ZERO
BELLY
SMOOTHIES

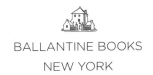

BALLANTINE BOOKS
NEW YORK

A Ballantine Books Trade Paperback Original

Copyright © 2016 by David Zinczenko

Published in the United States by Ballantine Books, an imprint of Random House, a division of Penguin Random House LLC, New York.

BALLANTINE and the HOUSE colophon are registered trademarks of Penguin Random House LLC.

ISBN 978-0-399-17844-3
ebook ISBN 978-0-399-59392-5

Printed in the United States of America on acid-free paper

randomhousebooks.com

2 4 6 8 9 7 5 3 1

Design by George Karabotsos
with Laura White
Photographs by Jeff Harris

DAVID ZINCZENKO

ZERO BELLY

SMOOTHIES

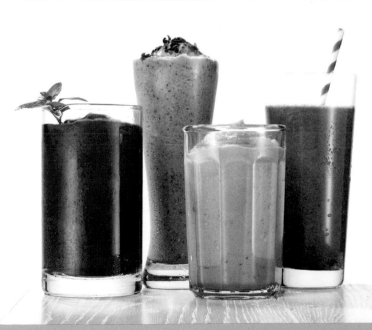

✳ CONTENTS

✱ INTRODUCTION
SHAKE OFF

If you had the power to make your life better with the push of a button, would you use it?

Well, that power is yours. With one simple whir, you can turn your body into a hyper-efficient fat-burning machine by revving up your metabolism, toning and defining your muscles, and turning off the genes that contribute to fat storage and myriad chronic health issues.

All you need is a blender, and the recipes in this book.

THE WEIGHT!

Zero Belly Smoothies are plant-based protein drinks that have been shown to make a dramatic impact on people's lives in as little as 72 hours. They will flatten your belly, heal your digestive system and strip away unwanted fat in just days. All you need to do is blend them up and drink them down.

I know these smoothies will work for you, and fast, because I've seen them work for so many others. Consider the case of Fred Sparks. A 39-year-old emergency-response advisor from Katy, Texas, Fred used *Zero Belly Smoothies* as part of his weight-loss program. "I noticed results in the first week," he says. "It really was amazing." Fred lost 21 pounds and 5 inches off his waist in just the next six weeks.

Martha Chesler, 52, who lost 21 pounds and 7 inches off her waist in less than 40 days, had the same experience:

"I saw results immediately." she says. In fact, our original *Zero Belly* Test Panel of more than 500 men and women lost as much as 3 inches off their waist in less than a week, and 16 pounds in the first 14 days. Now, you can achieve results like these even more quickly, with this carefully created, highly effective sample of the delicious drinks you'll find in *Zero Belly Smoothies.*

What's So Special About Smoothies?

They are fast, effective, simple to whip up, and delicious, which makes them ideal for a weight loss program. Consider the proof:

In a 2012 study in *Current Nutrition and Food Science,* researchers put a group of obese adults on a regimen in which they replaced breakfast and dinner with a high-protein smoothie. That was all: no exercise, no limit on what else they could eat. After 12 weeks, the subjects lost up to 18.5 pounds and reported significant improvements in "physical functioning, general health, vitality, and mental health."

A high-protein diet featuring meal-replacement drinks is more effective than exercise at helping people lose weight and keep it off, according to a 2013 meta-analysis of 20 studies in *The American Journal of Clinical Nutrition.*

Five percent of your body weight is the gold standard to prove effectiveness in a weight-loss plan. But smoothie-based plans beat that number consistently. In a study at the University of Kentucky in 2009, patients were asked to drink at least 3 smoothies a day. After 18 weeks, the subjects lost an average of 16.4 percent of their body weight—up to 44 pounds!

When researchers at Columbia University crunched the numbers on six separate studies following dieters on either a smoothie-based plan (one or two smoothies a day) or a reduced-calorie plan, they found that both sets lost weight, but those on the smoothie-based plan experienced "significantly greater weight loss" at both the 3-month and 1-year marks. In a 2015 review of studies on weight-loss plans, researchers at Johns Hopkins reported that participants who used low-calorie meal-replacement drinks like smoothies lost more weight than other dieters over the course of 4 to 6 months.

Are you ready to make the magic work for you?

It Worked for Her!

I've been amazed and gratified at how Zero Belly has changed the lives of thousands of Americans. Before going on the plan, Jennie Joshi would avoid walking past the full-length mirror in her Morristown, NJ home. "I hated the way I looked. I wanted to see the old me," says the mother of two.

Anyone who has had a child knows that feeling and how difficult it can be to lose pregnancy weight. A University of Chicago study last year found that 75 percent of moms were heavier than they were pre-pregnancy a year after giving birth and 45 percent had retained more than 10 pounds.

A high-risk pregnancy made it impossible for Joshi to exercise; she even had to limit her walking. Her weight gain was more than she had expected, and she struggled to lose it. "I really wanted to get rid of my belly," she says. But the calorie-cutting diet programs weren't doing it for her; then she learned about the *Zero Belly Diet* and signed up as one of the program's first test panelists. She was drawn to its no-sacrifice approach: "I loved that I could just focus on eating healthy foods and not worry about controlling portions."

She says the healthy recipes in the book made the difference because they included family-friendly options that even a foodie like her husband would enjoy. "Unlike a fad diet that you do once and stop, it's a lifestyle that's easy to make your own," she says.

Joshi also followed the program's suggested workouts and mixed in some running, spinning, and Zumba. In just four weeks, she lost 11 pounds.

"I saw the pregnancy pooch leaving," she says, and she pressed on, eventually dropping 26 pounds and fitting into a size 4 dress.

Her co-workers were astonished. "They wanted to know what I was doing."

What she was doing was drinking Zero Belly Smoothies.

And It'll Work for You!

One of the key components in Zero Belly Smoothies is the veggie protein powder and use of nut or dairy-free milks. Unless you've been living in an igloo for the past two decades, you should know by now that Americans do not eat enough fruits and vegetables. In fact, recent surveys have found that only about 30 percent of Americans are eating the recommended 5 or more servings of fruits and vegetables a day. That's a pretty pitiful performance and no doubt a partial cause of the obesity epidemic that grips this nation.

Another cause: Over the years, the line between smoothie and milkshake has been irrevocably blurred by the beverage industry. What was once a reliable, all-fruit concoction is now likely to be an ice-cream-and-added-sugar extravaganza, capable of carrying over 2,000 calories a serving (see Smoothie King, Hulk).

If you happen to be one of those 7 out of 10 of us who don't eat enough plant matter, then you need to make fast friends with Zero Belly Smoothies. They're the quickest, most delicious way to make up for the fruit-and-vegetable deficit, no ice cream required: Roll out of bed, toss some fruit in a blender, top with a bit of liquid, hit "liquefy." Boom! You're on the path to a skinnier, healthier you!

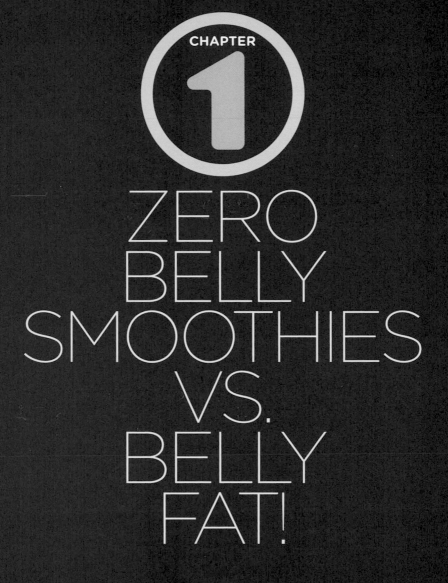

CHAPTER 1

ZERO BELLY SMOOTHIES VS. BELLY FAT!

Luke Skywalker has Darth Vader. Harry Potter has Lord Voldemort. Me, I have my own evil nemesis: I've made it part of my life's work to battle belly fat.

My battle started in junior high school. By the time I was 14, I was wrapped in a shame-inducing spare tire, carrying 212 pounds of high school huskiness on my 6-foot frame. Sure, I felt bad about being overweight. Sure, I was made fun of. Sure, I had trouble making friends and getting dates. But whenever life got me down, all I had to do was rip open another bag of Doritos and drown myself in fluorescent orange goodness or bum a ride to the mall and follow my nose to Cinnabon. Food was my refuge from feeling bad.

Then, at the still-young age of 52, my father passed away from a sudden, massive stroke. Always heavy since the time I was born, he had ballooned into obesity in the 1980s in much the same way I had. I was his son. I carried the same "fat genes" that he did.

Would this be my fate, too?

My father's death woke me up to the fact that excess weight—especially excess belly fat—was more than just a vanity issue. Belly fat may be the No. 1 cause of heart disease, stroke, diabetes, and cancer in America, and it contributes mightily to our epidemics of Alzheimer's, depression, and even inflammatory and autoimmune diseases. Indeed, new studies show that belly fat is utterly different from the other types of fat. It evolves out of a different set of stem cells than the fat found in other places on our bodies, its actions triggered by fat-storage genes that get turned on and cranked to high volume by our fast-food, high-stress lifestyle. Once those fat genes get turned on, visceral fat acts like an invading force, trying to take over our bodies.

What was clear to me was this: Belly fat killed my dad.

I was going to find a way to fight back.

That's how my odyssey to find smart solutions to belly fat began. And to be honest, I've actually had some success. I'm the co-creator of Eat This, Not That!, America's most respected source for information on restaurant and grocery-store foods, and I'm also the nutrition and wellness correspondent for ABC News. By spreading the word about the outrageous calorie counts and sneaky additives that lurk in our food, I feel like I've really made a difference. The Eat This, Not That! series of books and the daily news coverage on *EatThis.com* have helped hundreds of thousands of Americans lose tens of millions of pounds and changed the way we eat today.

But the war is only partly won. Two out of every three of us still struggle with belly fat, and the more we learn about it, the more the dangers of this scourge become apparent. We knew that belly fat, also known as visceral fat—the fat that's underneath your stomach muscles, wrapped around your internal organs—has biochemical functions that damage the human body, almost like a parasite intent on killing its host. But we knew little about how it operates, how it creates those chemicals, and what exactly they do to us. Until now.

Today, we know that fat storage is triggered, in great part, by a series of markers in our individual genetic codes. Some of us carry a number of genes linked to metabolic disorders like diabetes and obesity; others have a lower genetic propensity for these health issues. Once the "on" switch is flipped for our fat genes, we are at risk for weight gain and all the health issues that surround it—and no amount of exercise or calorie restriction is going to reverse that course completely. (That's why so many people who diet and work out like crazy still can't lose weight! Eureka!) And the No. 1 trigger for our fat genes is diet—especially a lack of certain nutrients.

We've also learned more about belly fat—how it's formed and how it behaves. A visceral fat cell is unlike any other kind of cell—fat cell or otherwise—in your body. Visceral fat doesn't even come from the same set of stem cells as other fat; it has evolved in an entirely different way. And as it gains greater purchase inside you, it spits out greater and greater levels of adipokines—a series of biochemical substances that do terrible things to your health. Adipokines raise your blood pressure, increasing your risk of stroke. They reduce your insulin sensitivity, leading to diabetes. They increase inflammation, which puts you at risk for everything from Alzheimer's to arthritis to psoriasis to cancer. They alter your hormonal response, eroding muscle tissue, increasing your risk of depression, and destroying your sex drive. They attack and scar your liver, leading to cirrhosis, cancer, and ultimately liver failure.

But in the past few years, this same research has given us several important breakthroughs—science that shows us how to finally master our midsections. And it's this new science that makes Zero Belly Smoothies so revolutionary. By making them with plant-based proteins and liquids, you'll tap the power of these foods to short-circuit your fat genes—turning off the parts of your DNA that trigger weight gain and activating your body to burn, not store, fat. Plus, the protein, fiber, and other nutrients in these creamy and satisfying drinks will boost your metabolism and dampen inflammation, leading to natural and sustainable weight loss. Drink these smoothies, and you'll build a lean, strong body and strip away unwanted belly fat without ever feeling hungry or deprived. The result: Weight loss will be easier, faster, more lasting, and (if I may say so myself) more delicious than you'd ever imagine.

FOUR WAYS SMOOTHIES MAKE LIFE EASIER

Focusing your weight-loss efforts on drinks will help you quickly strip away flab in a number of ways. Here's what makes Zero Belly Smoothies so effective:

1 They take the stress out of eating well.

A 2015 study at the Friedman School of Nutrition Science and Policy at Tufts University found that while most doctors subscribe to the notion of "all things in moderation," that long-standing bit of advice is actually wrong. When researchers looked at the diets of 6,814 people, they found that the more diverse the subjects' diets, the more likely they were to experience weight gain. In fact, those who ate the widest range of foods showed a 120 percent greater increase in waist circumference compared with those who had the least diversity. In other words, people who have the best success at weight loss pick a set number of foods and tend to stick to them. Zero Belly Smoothies allow you to do exactly that.

2 They make your workouts more effective.

Studies show that high-protein smoothies are highly effective at rushing nutrients to your muscles—which is why I recommend you have one of your two drinks immediately after exercise—and that blended fruit drinks, which include all the fiber, will actually keep you fuller longer than fruit juices. That means that your body can immediately begin healing the damage to your muscles caused by exercise. (It's the process of damage and repair that makes muscles grow stronger.) A 2013 review of studies in the *Journal of the International Society of Sports Nutrition* found that having a high-protein meal before and after exercise (with the meals not more than four hours apart) led to the best possible outcome for muscle building.

3 They crowd out the junk in your diet.

Perhaps you're thinking, "I already enjoy a protein smoothie. It goes by the name Muscle Milk, or Lean Body, or Met-Rx, or some other Very Serious Name, and it comes ready to drink! What makes your drinks any better?" Well, some of the most compelling research of the past few years has centered on how added sugars, particularly sugars in our beverages, can dramatically reshape our bodies and improve our health profiles. In a UCLA study of 54 overweight teens, individuals who reduced added-sugar intake by the equivalent of one can of soda per day over 16 weeks showed a reduction in belly fat and an improvement in insulin function. In a 2015 study in Sweden, researchers followed 42,400 men over the course of 12 years. They found that men who consumed at least two servings per day of sweetened beverages had a 23 percent higher risk of heart failure compared with those who did not. The impact is so great that you don't need to be meandering through middle age to see the impact: Even teenagers who consume food and beverages high in added sugars show evidence of risk factors for heart disease and diabetes in their blood, according to a study in *The Journal of Nutrition*. So why, then, would you drink something that contains maltodextrin, crystalline fructose, and sucralose (all forms of sugar); cellulose gum and gel (made from chemically digested wood chips); zinc oxide (also used in diaper rash medications); and 36 other ingredients—which is exactly what you get when you drink a container of Muscle Milk? Is this helping reduce your sugar intake and foster good gut health? Or does it make you afraid that one night the Toxic Avenger is going to crawl out of your belly button?

By stripping smoothies of the dairy, sugars, and artificial ingredients so common in popular shakes, Zero Belly Smoothies maximize all that's great about protein smoothies while zeroing out the negative. That means you'll be getting optimal nutrition in a delicious, easy-to-digest drink you can have at any point of the day—guaranteed to keep you full, shrink your belly, and leave you feeling full of energy. You'll discover the amazing and delicious recipes starting in Chapter Five.

4 They battle food allergies and reduce inflammation.

What's also unique about Zero Belly Smoothies is that they are vegan: no milk, no yogurt, no whey protein. A decade ago, when I wrote the *New York Times* best seller *The Abs Diet*, I had already become a fan of protein powders, and I recommended them from the start as a way of burning calories and building muscle. But that program centered on whey protein, and as more and more research points out the importance of gut health—and more and more people find themselves struggling with dairy-related digestion issues—I've discovered a much more belly-friendly alternative.

Plant-based protein powders are a low-sugar, high-fiber alternative to popular dairy-based supplements. I guzzled whey shakes for years and was astonished by how much lighter and leaner I felt when switching to a plant-based blend. A study by the University of Tampa that compared plant protein with whey found it to be equally as effective at changing body composition and boosting muscle recovery and growth. But with less sugar and a healthier fat profile, plant-based proteins will also improve your gut health at the same time as they're fueling your muscles. Hemp, rice, and pea proteins are all good options; however, you'll want to ensure you're getting a complete protein with a full amino acid profile, which is why a blend that combines all three is superior.

THE SIMPLE PATH TO ZERO BELLY

When you begin drinking Zero Belly Smoothies, you'll quickly put your weight-loss journey on autopilot. Here are the guidelines to keep in mind as you carve your own path to Zero Belly.

STEP 1

Ask Yourself Three Questions

When you build a smoothie, you need to be able to answer these three questions.

WHERE'S MY PROTEIN?
WHERE'S MY FIBER?
WHERE'S MY HEALTHY FAT?

Put together a drink that provides all three, and I guarantee you've got a line on a leaner, healthier body that's functioning at the peak of its genetic programming. Hitting all three in one sip means you're feeding your muscles; eating a slowly absorbed, hunger-controlling meal; maximizing the absorption of nutrients in your food to positively influence your genetics; and striking a major blow against cholesterol and elevated blood sugar. The Big Three will also help crowd out refined carbohydrates, saturated fats, added sugars, and additives. Here's the breakdown on these three key macronutrients:

PROTEIN.

Protein helps you burn fat in three ways. First, it's the building block of muscle, and you already know that muscle burns fat. Feeding your muscles helps them grow and fight back against the forces of fleshiness. Second, the very act of eating protein actually burns calories. It takes more than a kiss from a princess to turn a frog—or a cow, pig, or chicken, or a nut or bean, for that matter—into a human. As much as 20 to 35 percent of the calories you eat in the form of protein are burned up just digesting the protein itself. (Carbs and fat burn up no more than 5 to 15 percent of their calories.) And third, protein keeps you fuller longer—in part because that intense digestive process means your body perceives you as being satiated. In a 2013 study published in the journal *Appetite,* women were fed low-, moderate-, or high-protein afternoon snacks. Those who ate the most protein had the lowest levels of hunger and waited longer before they chose to eat again than those who ate lower-protein snacks.

Zero Belly Smoothies get their protein primarily from vegan protein powders, but oatmeal, spirulina powder, and nut butters are also excellent, smoothie-friendly sources.

FIBER.

Stop thinking about "good carbs" or "bad carbs" and start focusing on fiber. If you're eating fiber, you're packing your day with foods high in folate, vitamin B12, betaine, resveratrol, and sulforaphane—all critical nutrients that impact how active our fat-storage genes are. Fiber also allows the bacteria in your gut to produce the fatty acid butyrate, which influences the behavior of genes associated with insulin resistance and inflammation. Fruits, vegetables, grains, and nut butters all contribute fiber to my Zero Belly Smoothie recipes.

Fiber plays a number of additional roles in keeping us slim, but the most intriguing is its ability to suppress appetite. In spring 2014, an international team of researchers identified an anti-appetite molecule called acetate that's naturally released when fiber is digested. Acetate then travels to the brain, where it signals us to stop eating.

Some scientists believe that the dramatic reduction in fiber in our diets is perhaps the No. 1 factor in our obesity crisis. Professor Gary Frost from the Department of Medicine at Imperial College in London, who was part of the team that put together the acetate study, estimates that, thanks to food processing, the average Western citizen now eats about one-seventh as much fiber as humans did in the Stone Age. Makes you want to chew through a redwood, doesn't it?

HEALTHY FAT.

If you want to burn fat, you need to eat fat—regularly. A Zero Belly Smoothie needs to contain at least one of the following ingredients:

MONOUNSATURATED FATS: olives and olive oil, nuts (including peanuts) and nut butters, avocado, dark chocolate (at least 72 percent cacao)

POLYUNSATURATED FATS: sunflower seeds, sunflower oil, sesame seeds, pine nuts

PLANT-BASED SATURATED FATS: coconut (no sugar added), coconut oil (not hydrogenated)

OMEGA-3 FATTY ACIDS: flaxseeds, walnuts, chia seeds, hemp seeds

Though it may seem counterintuitive to add fat to a drink if you're trying to lose fat from your body, the fact is that eating a moderate portion of unsaturated fats, like the kind found in olive oil, avocados, and nuts, can ward off the munchies and keep you full by regulating hunger hormones. A study published in *Nutrition Journal* found that participants who ate half a fresh avocado with lunch reported a 40 percent decreased desire to eat for hours afterward. Moreover, increasing the amount of omega-3 fatty acids in your diet while reducing omega-6 fats (found in vegetable oil and foods fried in that oil) has proven to improve metabolic health and reduce inflammation.

STEP 2

Have a Zero Belly Smoothie Instead of a Meal or Snack

If your goal is to flatten your belly, then you need to maximize the amount of fat-burning, muscle-building, inflammation-fighting, gene-hacking nutrition that goes into your body every day.

These smoothies make that easy for several reasons. First, they're so delicious and easy to make that you can have them for breakfast, lunch, or dinner. Second, they ensure that you'll stay satiated and satisfied all day long. In a study presented at the North American Association for the Study of Obesity, researchers found that regularly drinking meal replacements increased a person's chance of losing weight and keeping it off longer than a year.

STEP 3

Make Smoothies Your Drink of Choice

If you're serious about shedding belly flab, I'd encourage you to cut out booze, soda, and any artificially sweetened drinks for the next few weeks. These drinks are loaded with sugars and artificial ingredients that can cause weight gain and bloating. Instead, switch to plain or carbonated water, and rely on a Zero Belly Smoothie when you want a sweet, satisfying drink. A 2015 study in the journal *Diabetologia* found that cutting just one sugary drink out of your day could lower your diabetes risk by up to 25 percent.

YOUR ZERO BELLY CHEAT SHEET

If you're already a fan of Zero Belly, then you know how effective it can be. Zero Belly Diet is the only program that attacks belly fat on a genetic level, reversing the action of your fat-storage genes even as it revs your metabolism and strips the junk from your diet. This collection of all-new drink recipes will expand your repertoire of simple, convenient, and delicious weight-loss shakes. But if you're new to the program, here's an at-a-glance guide to the Zero Belly principles, the diet plan that will flatten your belly, turn off your fat genes, and help keep you lean for life. (And if you would like a turbo-charged version of the program, check out the Zero Belly Smoothie Cleanse in Chapter Ten!)

SUBJECT: Number of meals

GUIDELINE: Three meals, one snack, and one Zero Belly Smoothie per day.

SUBJECT: The ZERO BELLY Foods

GUIDELINE: Each of the meals and snacks is build around the 9 ZERO BELLY Foods, each carefully selected for its micronutrient content. Every meal or snack should have protein, fiber, and healthy fat, derived from one of these sources:

Zero Belly Smoothies

Eggs

Red fruits

Olive oil and other healthy fats

Beans, rice, oats, and other healthy fiber

Extra plant protein

Leafy greens, green tea, and bright vegetables

Lean meats and fish

Your favorite spices and flavors (ginger, cinnamon, even chocolate)

SUBJECT: Portion size

GUIDELINE: While most diets center around controlling calorie intake, Zero Belly focuses on maximizing your intake of key nutrients. When you eat protein, fiber and healthy fat, you'll crowd much of the junk out of your diet, and control your hunger and calorie intake naturally.

SUBJECT: Secret Weapons

GUIDELINE: Smoothies. You hold in your hands the ultimate guide to Zero Belly Smoothies, and it's in these delicious drinks that the principles of Zero Belly come together so brilliantly. Each of the recipes in these books combines the Zero Belly foods into high-nutrient meals that are ready in just 90 seconds, and each combines protein, fiber and healthy fat to ensure you're always highly fueled and never hungry.

SUBJECT: Nutritional ingredients to emphasize

GUIDELINE: Protein, fiber, healthy fats

SUBJECT: Nutritional ingredients to limit

GUIDELINE: Dairy, wheat gluten, added sugars. (Note: Zero Belly is not strictly dairy-free or gluten-free. But because these can cause bloating and inflammation in some people, I've made sure that the entire program can be done without either ingredient. Each of the recipes in this book is gluten-free and dairy-free.)

SUBJECT: **Alcohol**

GUIDELINE: Limit yourself to no more than two or three drinks per week, to maximize the benefits of the program. Because of its high concentration of resveratrol, a compound that helps turn off fat-storage genes, red wine is the best choice

SUBJECT: **Exercise Program**

GUIDELINE: To turbocharge the weight-loss effects of Zero Belly, I've created the Zero Belly Workouts, an unique full-body fitness experience that builds abs while simultaneously toning your entire body. The complete Zero Belly Workout plan is found in Zero Belly Diet.

The Zero Belly Smoothie Matrix

The recipes in this book have been built by a team of dieticians and chefs to combine perfectly balanced nutrition with write-home-about-it flavor. But as always, experimenting with your favorite flavors to find the combination that works for you is part of the fun. And if you can find a recipe that truly sings to you, you'll be more likely to stick with it. More smoothies = more weight loss.

BASE

NUT MILK:
almond, hazelnut, coconut (unsweetened)

One of the key features of the smoothies in this book is that they're made primarily from plant sources. While milk and yogurt are great if you aren't sensitive to lactose, it seems that more and more people are recognizing that the bloating and discomfort they thought were normal parts of life are, in fact, reactions to lactose—the naturally occurring sugar in dairy products. Even if you have no issues with lactose that you know of, I urge you to try going vegan with your smoothies for the first two weeks. You may discover your belly has gotten magically flatter overnight.

Coconut water (unsweetened)

For a light smoothie, use unsweetened coconut water to up the liquid levels. You may soon find a daiquiri-flavored smoothie in your future.

Green tea

Add it to your smoothie, and green tea will shrink your belly. That's because green tea contains catechins, which trigger the release of fat from cells— particularly abdominal fat—then speed up the liver's capacity for turning that fat into energy. In a recent 12-week study, participants who drank four to five cups of green tea each day, then exercised for 25 minutes, lost an average of two more pounds than the non-tea-drinking exercisers!

FAT

NUT BUTTERS:
peanut, almond, cashew

Nut butters contain monounsaturated fats that will fill you up, not out. They contain fat-burning compounds that limit the amount of fat absorbed by the body, so some pass through undigested. They're also high in magnesium and B vitamins, which could lend you more energy to burn at the gym. They're also high in protein and fiber, which will make your smoothie more satisfying.

Coconut pieces or coconut oil

Because of its neutral flavor, coconut oil is an ideal mix-in for just about any smoothie you can think of— and if you're interested in torching belly fat, you'll start brainstorming. Consuming coconut oil reduces abdominal obesity, a study printed in the journal *Lipids* found. Half the study participants ate two tablespoons of coconut oil daily; the other half were given soybean oil. Only those in the coconut-oil group saw their waistlines shrink.

NUT OILS:
flax, walnut, hazelnut, peanut, almond

Always make sure there's some fat in your smoothie so that you're assured of staying satiated for several hours afterward. A teaspoon of any of these oils will give your smoothie a rich consistency and nutty flavor that you'll find truly satisfying.

Avocado

High in healthy monounsaturated fats, avocados also deliver a surprising dose of protein—2 grams per half a fruit. A study in *Nutrition Journal* found that participants who ate half a fresh avocado with lunch reported a 40 percent decreased desire to eat for hours afterward.

PROTEIN
Vegan protein powder

Supplementing your smoothie with protein powder is excellent for satiety, not to mention supporting the lean muscle that enables you to burn more fat. In a 2015 study in the *American Journal of Physiology—Endocrinology and Metabolism*, researchers found that those who ate twice as much protein as the Recommended Dietary Allowance had greater net protein balance and muscle protein synthesis—in other words, it was easier for them to maintain and build muscle, and hence keep their metabolisms revving on high. So even if you eat a burger for lunch and a couple of pork chops for dinner, you're still coming up short in the protein department. For your smoothie, you're best off with plant-based protein; whey, casein, and other dairy-based powders can cause bloating. Look for a product that has no artificial colors, sweeteners, or flavors. While hemp, rice, and pea proteins are all good options, you can ensure you're getting a complete protein with a full amino acid profile by getting a vegan protein blend that combines all three.

NUT BUTTERS:
peanut, almond, cashew

All of these provide healthy fats, fiber, and protein. But the king nut when it comes to protein is the humble peanut. In fact, ¼ cup of peanuts tops pecans (2.5 grams), cashews (5 grams), and even almonds (8 grams) in the protein power rankings. And they contain the mood-boosting vitamin folate.

Quinoa or oatmeal

In addition to its 4 grams of belly-filling fiber, a cup of oatmeal delivers as much protein as an egg. And quinoa is one of the few plant foods that offer a complete set of amino acids, meaning it can be converted directly into muscle by the body.

Spirulina

Spirulina is a blue-green algae that's typically dried and sold in powdered form, although you can also buy spirulina flakes and tablets. Dried spirulina is about 60 percent protein, and, like quinoa, it's a complete protein, meaning it can be converted directly into muscle in the body. A tablespoon delivers 8 grams of metabolism-boosting protein for just 43 calories, plus half a day's allotment of vitamin B12. It's a great option if a blended vegan protein isn't available.

Pomegranate or passion fruit

You may not think of fruit when you think of protein, but pomegranates stand out as protein powerhouses. The reason: The protein is stored in the seeds of the fruit. And pomegranate brings with it plenty of other powers as well: Research published in the *International Journal of Obesity* found that the anthocyanins, tannins, and high levels of antioxidants in pomegranates can help fight obesity. Like pomegranate, passion fruit delivers a surprising dose of protein thanks to its edible seeds; a half-cup also gives you 12 grams of fiber and more than half a day's vitamin C. Don't make the mistake of thinking that Pom Wonderful will give you the same benefits—it's full of sugars.

FIBER

Flax meal

Fiber-packed flaxseed contains more inflammation-fighting omega-3 fatty acids than other fat sources. That means it's good for reducing inflammation: Adding some ground flaxseed to your smoothie can help with muscle recovery. Flaxseed is highly sensitive and easily oxidized, so for the most health benefit, buy whole flaxseed and grind it just before adding to your smoothie. Two tablespoons gives you 2 grams of muscle-building protein as well as 4 grams of metabolism-enhancing fiber.

Oats

A tasty source of dietary fiber as well as protein. But that's not the only reason oats deserve a spot in your weight-loss shakes: Beta-glucans, part of the soluble fiber in oats, have been shown to lower total blood cholesterol and low-density lipoprotein (LDL) levels—meaning they can reduce your risk of heart disease.

Chia seeds

Not only are chia seeds packed with fiber and protein, helping keep you feeling full and satisfied—they also absorb toxins from your digestive tract. Though you can add a tablespoon of chia seeds directly into your blender, you'll get more goodness out of them—and add to the smoothness of your smoothie—by combining them with water so that they form a gel. Combine equal parts chia seeds and water in a container. The gel will keep in the fridge for a few weeks, so you can experiment with how much to add to your shakes.

Fruits and vegetables

Any fruit or vegetable will add fiber, but they're so important that I've given them their own special place at the table.

FRUITS AND VEGETABLES

Beets

Beets have a high nitrate content, and that's a big part of why you should be throwing them into your smoothies. They're thought to improve athletic performance (and working out ought to be a part of any weight-loss or weight-maintenance plan). Scientists looked at the performance of two groups of runners: one of individuals who consumed baked beets before a 5K run, and the second consisting of people who took a placebo before running the same distance. The beet eaters ran faster but didn't feel as if they were putting in extra effort!

Citrus fruits

Aside from packing a hefty amount of vitamin C, citrus fruits like oranges, lemons, limes, and grape-fruit contain plenty of folate, which helps produce and maintain your body's cells, and fiber, which is great for weight loss. They'll also add a zesty note to whatever else you're blending. Plenty of studies have shown that grapefruit stands alone as a particularly powerful weight-loss food. One study in the *Journal of Medical Food* found that people who ate half a fresh grapefruit a day lost 3½ pounds in 12 weeks despite making no changes in diet or exercise.

Pumpkins

These big, round, scary squashes deliver a powerful dose of vitamin A and harbor a secret stash of metabolism-boosting protein.

Leafy greens

If you like green juices, it's time to upgrade. Blenders preserve the satiating fiber that juicers press out. (And if you've tried using both at home, you know that cleaning a juicer is a special kind of hell.) Although you can't go wrong with the omnipresent kale, spinach is especially powerful when it comes to weight loss. In one Swedish study, 19 overweight women drank a mixture with 5 grams of spinach extract each morning. After three months, they lost 11 pounds, far more than the control group. The women also reported fewer food cravings, thanks to elevated levels of GLP-1, a physiological regulator of appetite and food intake. Feel free to pack your blender with plenty of leafy greens: Their high fiber and water content means that these low-density foods will have you feeling fuller, faster.

Stone fruits

New studies by Texas AgriLife Research suggests that plums, peaches, and nectarines may help ward off metabolic syndrome—a fancy name for the combination of belly fat, high cholesterol, and insulin resistance. And calorie for calorie, apricots contain more potassium than even bananas, the food source most commonly linked with this important element. Dietary potassium lowers blood pressure by reducing the adverse effects of sodium, including water retention.

Berries

Resveratrol is a heart-protecting antioxidant that people trot out to justify their Two Buck Chuck habit. But resveratrol is also found in red and purple berries before they go through the fermentation process. By adding berries to your smoothie, you'll benefit from compounds that can help reduce blood pressure and cardiac hypertrophy, lower levels of LDL (bad) cholesterol, and slow the progression of atherosclerosis (or hardening) of the arteries. All of which are highly beneficial to your mission of losing weight and keeping it off. In an animal study at the University of Michigan, researchers found that rats that ate a blueberry-rich diet for three months had significantly reduced belly fat.

Watermelon

Research at the University of Kentucky showed that eating watermelon may improve lipid profiles and lower fat accumulation.

BOOSTS

Ginger

I can't confirm whether Confucius had a six-pack (or suffered from a chronically queasy tummy), but legend has it the Chinese philosopher ate ginger with every meal. And now there's science to suggest that ginger can improve a number of gastrointestinal symptoms. In addition to curing bellyache, ginger may have a unique ability to accelerate gastric emptying, a study printed in the *Journal of Gastro enterology and Hematology* suggests.

Cayenne

Throw an impressive curveball at your next brunch by whipping up some virgin Bloody Mary smoothies, extra spicy, and burn off the dietary sins of the night before. Capsaicin, the natural compound that gives chili peppers that beautiful burn, has been proven to reduce belly fat, suppress appetite, and kick-start the body's ability to burn food as energy. Daily consumption improved belly-fat loss, a study published in *The American Journal of Clinical Nutrition* found.

Wheatgrass

What doesn't wheatgrass offer for a mere 30 calories? Even a tiny dose like this packs fiber, protein, tons of vitamin A and K, folic acid, manganese, iodine, and chlorophyll, to name a few. You don't need to know what each nutrient does for you; just know that a single tablespoon of wheatgrass will have you operating at peak performance levels.

Cocoa powder

Mix some cocoa powder into your smoothie for a boost of more than just flavor. In addition to delivering a gram of protein for every 12 calories, it will also give you 4 grams of fat-burning fiber and 20 percent of your daily value for the essential muscle-making mineral manganese.

Cinnamon

One of the best spices for weight loss, cinnamon also contains those magical polyphenols, which have been proven to slim bloated bodies and improve insulin sensitivity. A study published in *Archives of Biochemistry and Biophysics* showed that the consumption of cinnamon led to reduced belly fat in animals. And a series of studies printed in *The American Journal of Clinical Nutrition* found that adding a teaspoon of cinnamon to a carb-heavy meal could help stabilize blood sugar, preventing munchie-inducing insulin spikes.

Fresh mint or basil

Adding fresh herbs to smoothies is a little trick that yields big results. Basil pairs well with strawberries and watermelon, while mint works wonders on melon, blueberries, and papaya.

Honey

Remember that added sugar in any form—and that includes "natural" sugars like honey, maple syrup, or agave—is going to cut the healthfulness of your smoothie. As long as you're using fresh or frozen fruit, you shouldn't need added sugar. But if you do, honey at least gives you something in return, namely a host of phytochemicals that have antiviral and antibacterial properties.

Matcha powder

A powdered form of green tea, matcha delivers all the health benefits of tea in concentrated form.

Turmeric

Add it in powdered form, or find some fresh at the farmer's market, then peel, slice, and freeze it for easy smoothie use. The compound curcumin, found in turmeric, is a powerful anti-inflammatory that helps reduce the action of genes involved in belly-fat storage.

Fish oil

Fish oil has been canonized by hordes of wide-eyed nutritionists over the years, but the case for its sainthood sure is compelling. The tide of omega-3 fatty acids found in fish oil (usually made from fatty fish like salmon and sardines) may be the most versatile nutritional weapon out there, known to help protect the heart, fight inflammation, boost the brain, and reduce blood pressure, among other things. Look for a brand with a subtle flavor that will add all the nutritional punch without leaving your smoothie tasting like a can of sardines. I like Carlson Fish Oil liquids.

Fiber powder

Often sold under the name "psyllium husk" (for the seeds this powder is ground from), a dose of fiber is going to do more than promote a healthy colon. Fiber will slow the digestion of the smoothie in your stomach, which means not only will you stay fuller longer but also the sugar from the fruit will have a less dramatic impact on your blood sugar levels. And if the Quaker Oats dude has taught us anything, it's that fiber promotes a healthy heart as well.

ZERO BELLY SECRET:

FROZEN BANANAS

Not only do frozen bananas provide a luxurious creaminess and natural sweetness to your Zero Belly Smoothies, adding a texture similar to ice cream for a fraction of the calories (one medium banana contains only 106), but they also offer major weight-loss benefits. High in resistant starch, bananas do a great job of feeding the healthy gut bacteria that reduce bloating and help flatten your belly fast. A study found that women who ate a banana twice daily before meals for two months reduced belly bloat by 50 percent. Bananas are packed with potassium, which can reduce water retention. And they're a good source of fiber, which will keep you feeling full. Better yet, they're a cinch to prepare. I recommend freezing 10 to 12 at the beginning of each week.

Carefully peel the banana so that it stays intact. (Do not make the mistake of freezing the banana with the peel on!) Discard the peel and cut each banana in half.

Place up to 12 peeled banana halves into a resealable plastic freezer bag. Remove the air from the bag and seal tightly.

The bananas will keep in the freezer for a few months. When you're ready to blend, remove the bag from the freezer and grab the amount of bananas needed.

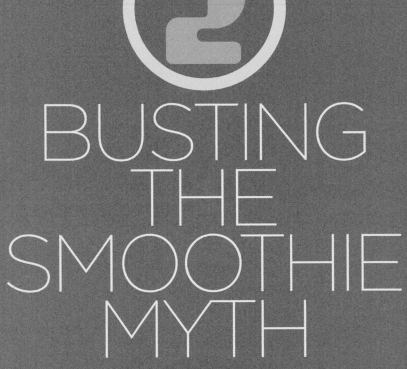

CHAPTER 2

BUSTING THE SMOOTHIE MYTH

Discover how not all Green Goddesses are good for you.

Why do you need a book of smoothie recipes, when there are smoothies for sale everywhere? It's a legit question. After all, just a few years ago you'd need to go to a specialty juice joint if you wanted a freshly blended smoothie. Now you can get them everywhere from Dunkin' Donuts to McDonald's. With so many healthy, fresh smoothies on the market, who needs to bother with blending her own?

Anyone who doesn't want to gain a lot of weight, that's who.

It's unfortunate, but most of the smoothies you'll find on restaurant menus nowadays are devious attempts to claim the halo of healthy, even as the drinks themselves pack a relentless attack of sugar. Consider:

At McDonald's, a small Blueberry Pomegranate Smoothie will give you 220 calories and 44 grams of sugar. A gram of sugar contains about 4 calories, which means 80 percent of those 220 calories come from sugar, while you're getting a mere 2 grams of protein. At Dunkin', the situation is even worse. Its Tropical Mango Smoothie is made of the following ingredients: water, yogurt, skim milk, milk, sugar, and less than 2 percent of everything else. The result is 260 calories, but 200 of those come from sugar.

I know what you're thinking: That's fast-food territory; of course their smoothies are unhealthy. Unfortunately, you won't do much better at the smoothie joint. In fact, you could do a whole lot worse.

For example, a Strawberry Surf Rider sounds pretty good for you; it's got berries, and it's got that healthy surfer vibe. This Jamba Juice classic combines strawberries and peaches with lemonade and lime sherbet, and it's gluten-free, with no artificial preservatives and no high-fructose corn syrup. So how good for you is it?

Well, how good for you is surfing with sharks if you don't know how to swim? The large Surf Rider packs 590 calories and a stunning 128 grams of sugar. You'd need to eat 20 Chocolate Creme Oreos to get that much sugar!

At Smoothie King, there's a whole "Fitness Blends" menu. But most of those Fitness Blends pack insane calorie counts: Consider the Hulk, the strawberry version of which contains 964 calories (more than half of what an adult woman should consume in a day) and four times as much sugar as protein. Its 88 grams of sweet stuff is what you'd get in about 3 cups of Breyers Black Raspberry Chocolate ice cream. (Even Smoothie King's Slim Blends can contain as much as 76 grams of sugar.)

Red Mango doesn't fare much better: Its Honey Badger Fat Burner sure sounds like it will help flatten your belly. But how does this drink burn fat when it contains 590 calories and 102 grams of sugar? (That's 3½ bags of M&Ms!)

HOW TO DECODE A SMOOTHIE

The truth is, most commercial smoothies are bad for you. And that's true of what you'll find not only in most restaurants but also on the grocery store shelves. For example, Bolthouse Farms offers an Amazing Mango Smoothie that packs 323 calories and 60 grams of sugar. That's not a smoothie, that's a dessert. A mere 3.1 fluid ounces of Dannon DanActive Blueberry packs 80 calories, which makes this drink twice as calorie-dense as a can of Mountain Dew. To assess a smoothie, make sure it meets the following criteria:

No added sugar.

All the sugar in your smoothie should come from the fruit used in the recipe. Beverages are the No. 1 source of added sugars in the American diet, and smoothies are no exception. Added sugar is the No. 1 cause of diabetes in America, and it has been linked to everything from heart disease to dementia. Sugar, corn syrup, maple syrup, agave nectar, honey—no matter how natural it might sound, you don't need it.

No juice.

The advantage a smoothie has over juice is that it contains all the fiber of the original fruit. But to cut corners, many smoothie makers use apple, orange, grapefruit, or pineapple juice as a base. While those are better than sugar water, they're not the foundation of a healthy smoothie.

At least 3 grams of fiber.

More is better, and if your smoothie is on the low side, consider asking for a boost of flax, chia, or psyllium to up the fiber count. Fiber slows the progression of sugar through the body; it's fast sugar that leads to abdominal fat.

At least 8 grams of protein.

A smoothie without protein isn't a smoothie, it's a juice—even if it has no added sugar and plenty of fiber. Protein is essential to feeding your muscles and increasing your metabolism, two goals of every smoothie you drink. And while protein smoothies are slightly higher in calories, those are calories that are actually worth drinking. Greek yogurt, nut butters, or a protein blend should get that puppy up on its feet.

A source of fat.

If your smoothie includes full-fat or 2 percent dairy, or a nut butter of some kind, or even flax or chia seeds, then you've got a healthy fat. Smoothies that don't include these, or which use fat-free ingredients, won't give you the fat-burning advantages you're looking for.

6 WAYS TO LOSE WEIGHT BEFORE NOON

Are you a morning person? Well, if you're carrying a few extra pounds around your middle, then probably not.

Turns out, morning people aren't just happier than night owls, they're lighter, leaner, and healthier, too. And it's not just getting up early that keeps them trim—though, more on that to come. There are a number of things you can do in the first half of the day that will nix the munchies, boost your metabolism, and turbocharge your weight loss—all before noon.

1
CATCH THE WORM

Early birds may catch the worms, but they don't overeat them. Or so suggests a recent study from Northwestern Medicine that found late sleepers—those who woke at about 10:45 a.m.—took in 248 more calories a day, ate half as many fruits and vegetables, and consumed twice the fast food of those who set the alarm clock earlier. A second study by researchers from the University of Roehampton found that morning people—those who leap out of bed at 6:58 a.m.—were generally healthier, thinner, and happier than the night owls, who start their day at 8:54 a.m. Coax yourself into waking up early by gradually setting your smartphone's alarm clock 15 minutes earlier every week, and wake up to a slimmer you.

2
GET SOME NOOKY

A little sexy time before rush hour can trigger the release of oxytocin, a hormone naturally released during times of bonding, including sex, that research shows can minimize stress hormones and suppress the appetite. According to a study in the journal *Aging,* daily injections of oxytocin—dubbed "the love hormone"—reduced the amount of food animals consumed, as well as abdominal fat and body weight, during and for nine days following the 17-day treatment. Other research suggests oxytocin and cortisol— the major stress hormone—are inversely related. As one goes up, the other goes down. That's good news for your waistline, as elevated cortisol can increase your appetite and cause weight gain. If you're a mom or dad, there's even more reason to linger in bed: A study in the journal *Psychoneuroendocrinology* showed parents' stress levels are 30 percent higher with the early-morning breakfast-before-the-school-bus rush and peak at about 8:15 a.m.—about the time they head out the door.

3
DO THE SUN DANCE

Roll out of bed and, before you do anything else, open all the blinds. According to a study published in the journal *PLOS ONE,* people who had most of their daily exposure to bright light in the morning had a significantly lower body mass index (BMI) than those who had most of their light exposure late in the day—regardless of how much they ate. Researches say 20 to 30 minutes of morning light is enough to affect BMI, and even dim light with just half the intensity of sunlight on a cloudy day will do. According to study authors, morning rays help synchronize the body's internal clock that regulates circadian rhythms and metabolism. Just put your clothes on first.

4
DO BRUNCH INSTEAD

How can Sunday's lazy-morning routine keep you slim? No, it's not the cartoons. Not the pj's. It's the shift in your eating habits to later in the day. Nighttime fasting—or simply eating breakfast later than normal to reduce your "eating window"—may boost your body's ability to burn fat as energy, according to a study in the journal *Cell Metabolism.* Researchers put groups of mice on a high-fat, high-calorie diet for 100 days. Half the mice were allowed to nibble throughout the night and day on a healthy, controlled diet, while the others had access to food for only eight hours but could eat whatever they wanted. The result of the 16-hour food ban? The fasting mice stayed lean, while the mice that noshed round the clock became obese—even though both groups consumed the same amount of calories. Some fasting protocols are more aggressive than others, but 12 hours without food is enough for most people to enter into a fasted state, according to some experts. So make every day Sunday Funday and postpone breakfast by a few hours. Your skinny jeans will thank you.

5
SNACK *AFTER* LUNCH

A study published in the *Journal of the American Dietetic Association* found that midmorning snackers tend to eat more throughout the day than afternoon snackers. Researchers found that dieters with the midmorning munchies lost an average of 7 percent of their total body weight, while those who did not snack before lunch lost more than 11 percent of their body weight. That's a difference of nearly 6.5 pounds for a 160-pound woman with a weight-loss goal. Moreover, afternoon snacking was associated with a slightly higher intake of filling fiber and fruits and vegetables.

WALK IT OUT

Getting your heart rate up in the morning can zap calories, but one benefit of early a.m. exercise comes at night. That's because working out early in the day can help you get quality sleep—an essential and often overlooked component of successful dieting. In fact, new research suggests subpar sleep could undermine weight loss by as much as 55 percent! In one study, participants who added 45 minutes of moderate walking five times a week to their weekly routines reported 70 percent better sleep; and women whose gentle exercise routines consisted of three 15- to 30-minute stretching sessions per week saw a 30 percent improvement. Unlike afternoon and evening exercise that can rile us up before bed, researchers say morning exercise helps sync our natural circadian rhythms, which can also support the metabolism. For an extra boost, try sneaking in your workout before breakfast. According to some studies, exercising in a fasted state can burn almost 20 percent more fat compared with exercising with fuel in the tank.

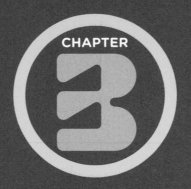

CHAPTER

3

HOW ZERO BELLY SMOOTHIES SMOOTH OUT YOUR BELLY

Learn how to heal your digestive system with one simple sip.

Have you ever experienced a gut feeling that something wasn't right? We might call it intuition or a sixth sense, and we might dismiss those feelings as completely illegitimate—just because you have a feeling in your belly doesn't mean there's logic involved.

But that thought process is actually wrong. What we interpret as gut feelings is actually the work of the enteric nervous system, a series of nerves and synapses that's just as complicated as the system in your brain. In fact, most of your serotonin, the "feel good" brain hormone that modern antidepressants work on, is located in the gut, not in the head.

Why does this matter? Because a healthy body, and a healthy mind, start with a healthy gut. That's why I've designed Zero Belly Smoothies to work with your digestive system in a way that helps end tummy troubles, reduce inflammation, and eliminate bloating.

A healthy belly means a healthy belly biome. In fact, you have a whole ecosystem that's operating inside you. There are about a hundred times as many bugs—single-cell bacteria—in your digestive tract as there are human cells in your entire body. On a per capita basis, you're about 99 percent microbe. And what's happening in your gut determines what happens in pretty much every other area of your body and your life. Before you can reset your metabolism and turn off your fat genes, you need to balance your belly.

SMOOTHIES TO THE RESCUE!

The human GI tract contains more than 500 species of bacteria—trillions of microbes that help to break down food, while also playing a role in knocking off any invading bugs that might be taking a ride on your radicchio. In fact, some of the bacteria in your gut even help ward off the pathogens that cause colds and flus. But like any efficient military, your bug brigade needs solid leadership—otherwise, you get chaos and mutiny. A balanced gut means your squirming little squadron is working with maximum efficiency on your behalf. But when things get out of whack—because of a poor diet or, sometimes, medications like antibiotics and even heartburn remedies—the forces below your navel can turn on you. Studies show that obese people have higher levels of bad bacteria from the phylum Firmicutes, while lean people have higher levels of good bacteria from the phylum Bacteroidetes.

So it's important to help the good bacteria along, because the bad bacteria in your gut release toxins, which inflame the GI tract. As long as these bacteria are kept in check, that's not a problem. But when they begin to overwhelm the better-trained bacteria, those toxins begin to cause inflammation in your digestive tract—a condition known as "leaky gut." Essentially, think of your intestinal tract as a fine screen, with little tiny holes through which nutrients can move into the bloodstream from your food. When bacteria get out of whack, they begin to irritate the lining of the intestines, and those holes become larger. Bacteria, food particles, and other nasty things escape your GI tract and get into your bloodstream.

A leaky gut leads to inflammation, as pathogens begin to attack the body and the body fights back. That can trigger your fat-storage genes, leading you to gain more weight than someone eating the same amount of food and spending the same amount of time in the gym. In fact, it's the fatty acid butyrate, produced by healthy bacteria feasting on fiber, that helps dampen the behavior of genes linked directly to insulin resistance and inflammation. Less fiber means less healthy bacteria, which means less butyrate and, eventually, inflammation and diabetes.

That's why these smoothies are designed to restore your gut health. In one study, adults with "large visceral fat areas" who drank 7 ounces of bacteria-supporting liquids lost up to 9 percent visceral fat and 3 percent belly fat, while the control group lost nothing.

Bad bacteria in your gut feed off sugar, just like the bacteria in your mouth. That's why Zero Belly Smoothies are low in sugar and high in fiber: They starve the bad bugs and feed the good ones. In one Canadian study, subjects who were supplemented with a natural insoluble fiber not only lost weight but also reported less hunger than those who received a placebo. Researchers discovered that the subjects who received the fiber had higher levels of ghrelin—a hormone that controls hunger—and lower levels of blood sugar. The reason insoluble fiber works so well in balancing the gut is that it's not digested; it remains in your GI tract all the way to the end, reaching the good bacteria in the lower intestines and helping them fight off the bad guys.

My Zero Belly Smoothies are also high in omega-3 fatty acids, which help reduce inflammation, and gluten-free. Recent studies have found that gluten can negatively impact gut bacteria, even in people who are not gluten sensitive.

After reading all of this about belly bugs, you might be wondering: "How come I'm not eating yogurt all day long, or popping those probiotic supplements? Isn't that how you get those healthy gut bugs into your system?"

Well, yes. It's true that some yogurts contain beneficial bacteria that can send reinforcements into the gut when you need them. *Lactobacillus acidophilus* is the bacteria you want to look for, with yogurts that say "live active cultures." But most yogurts are so high in sugar that they do more to promote unhealthy gut bacteria than anything else, which is why I don't recommend it on the Zero Belly plan. And while probiotics may help, these supplements are unregulated, and it's not clear whether they pack enough bacterial cultures to make a difference. But relying on supplements and even yogurt isn't a great idea. It's like polluting a pond and then stocking it with fish. The new fish will eventually die, and then you'll have to ship in more fish. Wouldn't you rather have a healthy pond in which the natural aquatic life can live healthfully and thrive forever?

5 WEIRD THINGS THAT ARE KILLING YOUR HEALTHY GUT BUGS

Your belly is a war zone. Tribes of microbes battle it out every minute of every day in an epic clash that makes *Game of Thrones* look like *Wheel of Fortune*. Some of these gut bugs are good for you—they help digest food and create fatty acids that reduce inflammation and hinder fat storage. Others are less helpful; in fact, studies show that obese people have higher levels of unhealthy bacteria like *Staphylococcus* and Firmicutes, which cause inflammation and have been linked to an increased risk of diabetes.

One of the most powerful weight-loss effects of Zero Belly Smoothies is that they provide the healthy bacteria in your gut with plenty of fiber to munch on, helping them grow stronger, while reducing the amount of sugar in your diet. (Sugar is what the bad bacteria feed on.)

While experts are scrambling to figure out exactly what a "healthy" microbial community looks like, they've discovered that some of the things we're doing on a daily basis are giving a leg up to the bad-for-you bugs in our bellies. Here are five things that alter our gut microbes in unhealthy ways.

BAD BELLY MOVE #1

>Taking Antibiotics

Most people take antibiotics at least once a year. And while we know that antibiotics wreak havoc on bugs good and bad in your belly, the general theory among the medical community has always been that after you stop taking them, your body goes on to recover completely. But recent research reveals that broad-spectrum antibiotics leave lasting changes to the communities of microbes that live in us. Antibiotics reduce the diversity of our microbiome by killing off whole communities of microbes, selecting communities that have resistance to the antibiotics, and allowing harmful "opportunist" microbes to flourish in the wake of treatment, according to recent research published in *The Journal of Clinical Investigation*. Antibiotics can be lifesaving if used when truly necessary. But don't seek them out every time you get the sniffles.

BAD BELLY MOVE #2

>Searing Meat

When you cook meat at high temperatures, and that includes beef, pork, fish, or poultry, chemicals called heterocyclic amines (HCAs) are produced. According to a study in *Nutrition Journal,* increased intake of HCAs causes changes to our gut microbiota that increase our risk to colorectal cancer. Consider slow cookers or long, languid barbecues the healthier alternative to pan-frying or grilling.

BAD BELLY MOVE #3
>Spraying Roundup

A controversial study published in *Interdisciplinary Toxicology* attempted to make a connection between glyphosate (better known as the herbicide Roundup, used on GMO crops and many a suburban lawn) and disturbances in the gut microbiota that lead to celiac disease. While chemical-industry-backed experts were quick to point out the flaws in the study (of which there are a few), the question of whether pesticides alter gut microbes has been answered in animal studies. A German study in *Current Microbiology* found that glyphosate encourages the growth of harmful bacteria like *Salmonella* and *Clostridium botulinum,* while slashing beneficial bugs like *Bifidobacterium* and *Lactobacillus.*

BAD BELLY MOVE #4
>Traveling Across Time Zones

You're not the only one with jet lag: It turns out our gut microbes have circadian rhythms, too. A recent study in the journal *Cell* found that our gut microbes are just as affected by changes to our circadian clock as we are. When we shift our sleep/wake cycles our gut flora changes, and beneficial bacteria are replaced by the growth of bacteria that have been linked to obesity and metabolic disease.

BAD BELLY MOVE #5

>Moving North

Have you ever heard of Bergmann's rule? It says that body size increases with latitude. Well, a recent study in the journal *Biology Letters* found that the reason for this is that living in northern latitudes encourages the growth of Firmicutes microbes, which have been linked to weight gain, while decreasing microbes linked with slim body types called Bacteroidetes. The number of Firmicutes increases with latitude, and the number of Bacteroidetes decreases with latitude.

"GUT FEELINGS" THAT MAKE YOU FAT

How does belly fat feel?

If you said "squishy," "spongy," or the less elegant "gross," you may be right. But fat has other feelings associated with it, too: anxiousness, loneliness, even happiness sometimes. Because your belly doesn't exist in a vacuum. It influences, and is influenced by, a complex series of hormones that course through your brain and body constantly.

And those hormones not only drive our emotions but also are driven by them. Our bodies reflect our emotional state—our hearts pound when we're afraid, our blood pressure soars when we're angry, our stomachs churn when we're feeling guilty.

And our belly fat responds, too. Sometimes our emotion-driven hormones act directly on our fat cells, causing us to gain or lose fatty tissue. Other times they drive behaviors that lead to greater weight gain. Either way, being more in touch with your feelings can help you get more in touch with your abs. Here are the emotions that put your belly fat in motion.

FAT FEELING #1

>LONELINESS

Because It: **Messes up your hunger hormones**

Any bad mood can lead us to try to comfort ourselves with food, and loneliness is about as bad a feeling as you can have. But the link between loneliness and weight gain is more substantial than that. A new study in the journal *Hormones and Behavior* found that those who feel lonely experience greater circulating levels of the appetite-stimulating hormone ghrelin after they eat, causing them to feel hungrier sooner. Over time, folks who are perennially lonely simply take in more calories than those with stronger social support networks.

Break the Mood: Get off the computer. Use of social networks and high Internet use exacerbate feelings of loneliness. Go find people who share your interests, whether it's hiking, knitting, biking, reading, shopping, even eating.

FAT FEELING #2

>WEDDED BLISS

Because It: **Makes us copy our partner's bad habits**

A review of more than 600 studies found that being married, and transitioning into marriage, are both associated with weight gain.

Transitioning out of a marriage, however, is associated with weight loss. (Maybe that's how the quintuply divorced Billy Bob Thornton stays so slim.) The researchers found that weight gain occurs because of increased opportunities for eating due to shared, regular meals and larger portion sizes, as well as "decreased physical activity and a decline in weight maintenance for the purpose of attracting an intimate partner." That's science speak for "You let yourself go!"

Break the Mood: Assuming bliss isn't an emotion you want to give up on, the next best approach is to identify the shared habits that are harming your health. The best way to stick to a healthy diet and exercise routine is to do it with someone else. So partner up: Consider taking cooking classes and fitness classes together, and make weight loss a fun goal for the two of you.

FAT FEELING #3

>DEPRIVATION

Because It: **Manifests itself as hunger**

Food. Sex. Adventure. Validation. If you feel as if you or someone else is depriving you of something, then you are more likely to overeat, regardless of how "good" you want to be. And if it's food you're trying to resist, you'll also experience more cravings for whatever it is you aren't getting, according to a study in the *International Journal of Eating Disorders*. Our brains actually become wired to view forbidden foods as rewards, setting us up for cravings that are hard to satisfy. And this, my friends, is why most diets fail. You can resist chocolate cake for only so long before you find yourself at the diner, wolfing down three slices.

Break the Mood:

If you're feeling deprived by your diet, build in a cheat meal at least once a week in which you can indulge guilt-free. Doing this will help you avoid viewing certain foods as off-limits, which will help you crave them less.

FAT FEELING #4

>STRESS

Because It: **Triggers fat storage**

When stress hits, the first thing your body does is to up its production of adrenaline. Adrenaline causes fat cells all over your body to squirt their stores of fatty acids into your bloodstream, where they can be used as energy. This was great back when stress meant facing a charging saber-toothed tiger or an attacking horde of bar-barians, and you could turn and head for the hills. But you can't really run away from a deadline or take up arms against a traffic jam. All you can do is bear down and, to help soothe your nerves, maybe have a snack. And another. Meanwhile, a second hormone called cortisol grabs all those unused fatty acids from your bloodstream and stores them in your belly region. With that fat stored, not burned, your body goes looking for more calories to replace the fatty acids it released earlier (back when it thought the hordes were invading).

Break the Mood: Laughter is the best stress reliever. It lowers your heart rate, improves your mood, makes you friendlier, and decreases anxiety. So go to YouTube and plug in one of these search terms: "a bad lipreading of the NFL," "dogs just don't want to bathe," or the ever popular "grandmas smoking weed for the first time."

FAT FEELING #5

>BOREDOM

Because It: **Confuses your brain**

When you're bored you actually lose your ability to make smart food choices; you become an "emotional eater," according to a new study in the *Journal of Health Psychology*. And boredom turns you into the worse kind of emotional eater, because you not only make the wrong food choices but also eat much more of those fattening foods than you normally would. Unfortunately for us, "because I'm bored" is one of the top reasons people give when they're asked about their emotions before they eat.

Break the Mood: You feel bored when you are dissatisfied, restless, and unchallenged, according to a study in *Frontiers in Psychology*. The best way to beat boredom is to find something to do that is purposeful and challenging. Instead of trying to entertain yourself, look for opportunities to help others.

FAT FEELING #6

>ANXIOUSNESS

Because It: **Leads to disordered eating**

When you're anxious, your body feels like it's under a tremendous amount of stress all the time. This is why anxiety is a powerful trigger for weight gain. A recent study in the journal *Eating and Weight Disorders* placed anxiety as "one of the most important factors significantly associated with weight gain." In fact, two-thirds of people with eating disorders also suffer from anxiety, and the anxiety usually existed first.

Break the Mood: Two of the most proven cures for anxiety are exercise and spending time in nature. Combine both with an outdoor run or bike ride and race away from the anxiousness.

5-MINUTE FLAT-BELLY TIP:

BREW SOME GREEN TEA

Adding a cup (or two) of green tea to your daily regimen can help fire your fat furnace in two ways. First, it controls blood sugar and quashes hunger: In a Swedish study that looked at green tea's effect on hunger, researchers divided up participants into two groups: One group sipped water with their meals, and the other group drank green tea. Not only did tea sippers report less of a desire to eat their favorite foods (even two hours after sipping the brew), they found those foods to be less satisfying. And second, it boosts your calorie burn, especially if you have it before any type of exercise: In a recent 12-week study, participants who combined a daily habit of four to five cups of green tea each day with a 25-minute sweat session lost an average of two more pounds than the non-tea-drinking exercisers. It's the power of the unique catechins found in green tea that can blast adipose tissue by triggering the release of fat from fat cells (particularly in the belly), then speeding up the liver's capacity for turning that fat into energy. All this while doing something unique for your heart: A 2015 study from the Institute of Food Research found that the polyphenols in green tea block a "signaling molecule" called VEGF, which in the body can trigger both heart disease and cancer.

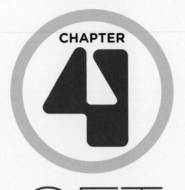

GET PREPARED!

Become a mix master with these easy steps.

—

There's a time machine in your kitchen. With the touch of a button, it will start whirring and spinning and altering the very nature of whatever goes inside of it. Solids will change into liquids; multiple types of complex organic matter will merge into a single, coherent power source.

Harness this power, and you can dramatically change your body in just 10 days—slowing the aging process and stripping away 10, 12, 14 pounds and up to 3 inches from your waist—without hunger, without deprivation, without ever feeling like you're sacrificing anything. In the process, you will literally alter your genetic profile, turning "off" the genes for fat storage and diabetes and making weight loss quick, effortless—automatic.

This time machine—your blender, of course—has probably been sitting on your counter, neglected, for years.

If you're like most Americans, you whip it out a couple of times each summer for daiquiris or margaritas or when the kids want a homemade milk shake. But if you want to truly take control of your weight, your health, and your life—if you want to lose belly fat quickly and keep it off forever—then you need to turn your blender into an everyday tool.

Here are a few rules to keep in mind as you explore the Zero Belly drinks:

Choose your protein.

As I mentioned earlier in this book, more and more studies are showing that vegetable proteins may have an even more powerful weight-loss effect than animal proteins. And because they're lactose-free and usually much lower in sugar, vegan proteins do a better job of fighting bloat and inflammation than traditional animal-based versions. Sorry, Miss Muffet, but we're skipping the curds and whey. Make sure your protein powder has at least 15 grams of protein per serving. While individual proteins like rice, hemp, or pea are fine, you're better off with a blended protein that gives you a full amino acid profile. (Note: I've left soy proteins off this list because highly concentrated doses of soy can have a negative impact on lean muscle tissue, thanks to the estrogen-like chemicals that occur naturally in the plant.) Here are some of the proteins I like the most:

VEGA ONE ALL-IN-ONE NUTRITIONAL SHAKE

A blend of vegan proteins, Vega gives you everything you need in one dose. Vega Sport Performance Protein will do the same.

1 scoop: 170 calories
6g fat (0g trans fat)
13g carbs
>1g sugar
20g protein

SUNWARRIOR WARRIOR BLEND RAW VEGAN PROTEIN With 19 grams of protein and 100 calories per serving, this organic protein is derived from peas, cranberries, and hemp, with no sugars, gluten, or artificial sweeteners to cause a metabolism-confusing midday crash. But it's tasty enough to take on its own. If you down some pre-workout, the branched-chain amino acids can give your gym session a boost.

1 scoop: 100 calories
2g fat (0g saturated fat)
2g carbs
0g sugar
19g protein

GARDEN OF LIFE RAW MEAL
This organic protein blend, good for a meal replacement, is derived from belly-fat-blasting brown rice, quinoa, and beans, plus tea and cinnamon extract. With 34 grams of protein and 10 grams of fiber per two-scoop serving, having one of these for lunch before a workout will keep you feeling full and energized while preserving muscle.

2 scoops: 155 calories
2.5g fat (1g saturated fat)
16g carbs
3.5g sugar
17g protein

ALIVE! ULTRA-SHAKE PEA PROTEIN
Pea protein is rich in amino acids and is easy to digest. While not as preferable as a full blend, this variety by Alive! contains a substantial 15 grams of protein per scoop, plus a multi-vitamin's worth of nutrients.

1 scoop: 120 calories
>1g fat (0g saturated fat)
15g carbs
9g sugar
15g protein

NUTIVA ORGANIC HEMP PROTEIN Stifle the Woody Harrelson jokes: Hemp protein is derived from the less-fun parts of the hemp plant, offering a substantial amount of fiber (here, 8 grams) that's easy to digest. With 15 grams of protein per scoop, this organic option is an ideal mix-in for oatmeal or smoothies (or brownies, if that's your thing); the fiber will make you feel fuller longer, and it contains eight essential amino acids to build muscle.

1 scoop: 90 calories
3g fat (0g saturated fat)
9g carbs
1g sugar
15g protein

Freeze!

Don't fall for the common misconception that you need to always use fresh fruit. Beyond being more affordable, the fruit you find in the freezer section is normally picked at the height of the season and flash-frozen. It also makes for colder, creamier smoothies. Simple rule of thumb: If a fruit is at the peak of its season, buy it fresh. If not, stick with frozen. (If you don't use frozen fruit, you can add a cube or two of ice to each recipe.) And don't forget to use the frozen bananas I told you about earlier in this book!

Mix up the milks.

Almond and coconut milk are commonly available in most markets, but don't hesitate to experiment with whatever nondairy milks are on hand at your local market: hazelnut, hemp, rice, and oat milk all can add a creamy dimension to any of these recipes. One to avoid: soy milk. Soy is particularly high in naturally occurring compounds called estrogenics, which raise estrogen levels and lower testosterone levels, promoting fat storage. That doesn't mean you need to avoid soy at all costs, but most Americans eat far more soy than they know. I've chosen to leave soy out of Zero Belly recipes for just these reasons.

Or mix in the teas.

Green tea makes a terrific base for a smoothie, because the active ingredient in green tea, EGCG, is an effective metabolism booster. And green tea is mild (unlike harsher black teas), so it makes for a great jumping-off point. White tea and rooibos are also great smoothie starters.

Boost your fiber.

While the Zero Belly Smoothies all have fiber as a component, you can make this program even more effective by adding additional fiber in the form of flax meal or psyllium husk. Fiber is a type of carbohydrate that makes up the structural material in the leaves, stems, and roots of vegetables, grains, and fruits. It's like the spine of plants. But unlike sugar and starch—two other types of carbs—fiber stays intact until it nears the end of your digestive tract. This is what makes fiber beneficial.

There are two basic types of fiber, and they have separate functions.

Insoluble fiber is found in wheat bran, nuts, and many vegetables. Its structure is thick and rough, and it won't dissolve in water, so it zips through your digestive tract and increases the bulk of your stool. (Definitely nothing sexy here.)

Soluble fiber is found in oats, beans, barley, and some fruits. It dissolves in water to form a gel-like material in your digestive tract. This allows it to slow the absorption of sugar into your bloodstream. What's more, soluble fiber, when eaten regularly, has been shown to slightly lower LDL (bad) cholesterol levels.

More fiber will mean a more satisfied you. In fact, while scientists have long known that eating fiber helps us control hunger, they didn't really understand why until 2014, when researchers at the Imperial College of London discovered an anti-appetite molecule called acetate. This molecule is released naturally when the healthy bacteria in our colon digests fiber. During the digestion process, the fiber ferments and releases a large amount of acetate as a waste product. Once created, the acetate travels from the colon to the liver and the heart and eventually winds up in the hypothalamus, the region of the brain that controls hunger. Once there, it causes the firing of specialized neurons that signal us to stop eating.

Pour first, then pile.

As you're building your smoothie, add liquids first, then protein and fruit to your blender. It's easier on the blender and gets things moving faster. For a thicker, spoonable smoothie, use less liquid than dictated by the recipe. Add more for a fruity, milk-like consistency.

Start slow.

Set your blender on a low speed and wait a few seconds, or until the larger pieces of fruit begin to break down, before you turn up the speed. Going all out at the start can cause air bubbles to form, which you'll then have to get in and pop (after turning the blender off, of course).

Buff up your blender.

The fact is, you need a quality blender in order to make quality smoothies. That old model from your dorm room won't be able to crush the ice and frozen fruit quickly enough, which means it can melt and ultimately dilute your precious creation rather than giving it that bracing, velvety texture you want. Here are some of the models I like:

CUISINART POWEREDGE 1,000-WATT BLENDER.

An easy-to-use and versatile blender that's great for everything from your fitness-minded smoothies to the kids' strawberry milk shakes.

KITCHENAID 5-SPEED DIAMOND BLENDER.

Does it all for a reasonable price.

KITCHENAID 5-SPEED HAND BLENDER.

If you travel a lot or like to mix it up in the office, this handy tool is a great solution.

MAGIC BULLET.

A small, handheld device that makes blending simple.

NINJA MASTER PREP.

A high-speed blender that won't take up a lot of room on your countertop.

NINJA ULTIMA BLENDER 244.

This professional-grade blender may be a bit more expensive, but it can muscle its way through just about any food and is easy to clean.

NUTRIBULLET.

Perfect for blending while traveling.

VITAMIX 5200.

Gorgeous, high-powered, and expensive. But worth it if you blend a lot and want to show off to your nosy friends.

Respect the ratio.

Once you learn the basic proportions of liquids to solids, you can turn anything into a drinkable smoothie. For every 3 cups of fruit or other solids, you'll need about 1 cup of liquid. Keep in mind that protein powders will thicken your drink.

Invest in a blender bottle.

Zero Belly Smoothies are best right out of the blender, because once you crush up a food, its nutrition starts to deteriorate rapidly. So if you want to take a Zero Belly Smoothie to travel, consider making it the night before and freezing it in a blender bottle. (Look for one with a metal mixer ball, which helps reblend the drink when you shake it.)

Mess around.

While each and every one of the recipes in this book will result in a fast, healthy, and unbelievably delicious smoothie, consider them simply a selection of bases to which you can add all varieties of nutritional enhancements. Find some fresh turmeric at the green market? Some weird new fruit down at Whole Foods? Or an interesting spice you haven't tasted before? Don't be afraid to look at each and every healthy food you see and think, "I wonder what that would taste like in a smoothie?"

Chances are, it'll taste delicious.

ST. PATRICK'S DAY EVERY DAY

Green tea—subtle and woodsy in flavor—makes a terrific base for smoothies, and it brings to the mix its own metabolism-boosting benefits. One study found that people who drink green tea daily have an average of 20 percent less body fat that non-tea-drinkers.

But if you're the adventurous type who's interested in taking weight loss to another level, you may want to explore the traditional Japanese green tea known as matcha. Matcha is a powdered green tea that some research indicates may be an even more potent weight-loss weapon. The concentration of EGCG—the super-potent nutrient found in green tea—may be as much as 137 times greater in powdered matcha tea. EGCG can simultaneously boost lipolysis (the breakdown of fat) and block adipogenesis (the formation of new fat cells).

One study found that men who drank green tea containing 136 milligrams of EGCG—what you'd find in a single 4-gram serving of matcha—lost twice as much weight than a placebo group and four times as much belly fat over the course of three months. And because the entire leaf is consumed, matcha also contains about 10 times as many antioxidants as regularly brewed green tea. Try blending a tablespoon of matcha into your smoothie.

THE TRUTH ABOUT OUR DRINKS

I f there's a single greatest secret to the effectiveness of Zero Belly Smoothies, it's this: When you're drinking a smoothie, you're not drinking one of the many other beverages on offer in America, most of which are, quite literally, toxic.

The average American now drinks about a gallon of soda a week. Add to that our odd new habits of swapping tap water for bottled "vitamin" water (120-plus calories) and giving up plain iced coffee for Mocha Frappuccinos (520-plus calories) and you can see how quickly the calories add up—and that's before chugging an "energy drink" (another 280 calories) that tastes exactly like what would happen if a crazed pastry chef hijacked a truckload of Smarties and drove it into a battery acid factory. Those three drinks alone give you 920 additional calories—almost half a day's worth!

In fact, liquid calories now make up a whopping 21 percent of our daily calorie intake—more than 400 calories every single day, more than twice as much as we drank 30 years ago. To give you a perspective on those numbers, imagine taking two slices of Pizza Hut Thin 'N Crispy Pepperoni Pizza, tossing them in a blender, and hitting "puree," then drinking the whole thing down. That's 420 calories. Now imagine that the typical American has been doing this every single day for years.

Wow. Disgusting, right?

But it's not just a story of calories in and calories out. More and more research is showing that the sugar in soda, energy drinks, iced teas, and commercial smoothies is literally attacking our bodies, causing the growth of belly fat and all the health crises that come with it. And one study found that sugar-sweetened beverages were responsible for more than 37 percent of the added sugars we consume every day. Here's what drinking those sweeteners is doing to us.

Added sugar causes your body to store fat around your belly.

Within 24 hours of eating fructose, your body is flooded with elevated levels of triglycerides. Does that sound bad? It is.

Triglycerides are the fatty deposits in your blood. Your liver makes them, because they're essential for building and repairing the tissues in your body. But when it's hit with high doses of sugar, the liver responds by pumping out more triglycerides; that's a signal to your body that it's time to store some abdominal fat.

Added sugar makes you skip going to the gym.

In one study at the University of Illinois, mice that were fed a diet that mimicked the standard American diet—i.e., one that was about 18 percent added sugars—gained more body fat even though they weren't fed more calories. One of the reasons was that the sugar-addled mice traveled about 20 percent less in their little cages than mice that weren't fed the sugary diet. They just naturally...slowed...down.

Added sugar is the No. 1 factor in your risk of dying from diabetes.

Researchers at the Mayo Clinic have come right out and said that added fructose—either as a constituent of table sugar or as the main component of high-fructose corn syrup—may be the No. 1 cause of diabetes and that cutting sugar alone could translate into a reduced number of diabetes deaths the world over.

Added sugar makes you dumb, demented, and depressed.

"Reduce fructose in your diet if you want to protect your brain," announced Fernando Gomez-Pinilla, professor at the University of California Los Angeles. He and his team tested how well rats recovering from brain injury learned new ways to get through a maze. They found that animals that drank HFCS took 30 percent more time to find the exit. "Our findings suggest that fructose disrupts plasticity—the creation of fresh pathways between brain cells that occurs when we learn or experience something new," he says.

That's pretty scary stuff, but behind that slightly sickening science comes some great news. Because if you want to strip away pounds, shrink your belly, and begin to sculpt a leaner, fitter body—while also boosting your health, calming your mind, and fighting back against some of the most significant diseases of our time—just changing what you drink could be all you need.

One study at Johns Hopkins University found that people who cut liquid calories from their diets lose more weight—and keep it off longer—than people who cut food calories. Simply cutting out liquid calories—by switching your usual drink to tea—could save you nearly 42 pounds this year alone!

But to make the Zero Belly Smoothies plan work, you first have to rid yourself of the liquid toxins your body has been piling up. Here's how to do it:

STEP 1

>Swear Off Sodas and Bottled Teas

Annual weight loss: 12 pounds

According to the National Institutes of Health, the third largest source of food calories in the American diet isn't a food at all. It's soda. We get more calories from soda every day than we do from meat, dairy, or anything other than baked goods. How can that be possible? Because of all the sugar. Mountain Dew, for example, not only delivers 52 grams of sugar per 12-ounce can but also gives you a delicious side helping of brominated vegetable oil, a component of rocket fuel. And I don't mean metaphorical rocket fuel—I mean the stuff they actually put in the engines to keep the gears from exploding.

STEP 2
>Don't Drink Juice Drinks

Annual weight loss: 19 pounds

If the FDA ever forces drink manufacturers to start properly labeling their products, SunnyD would have to be called ObesiD. (Some versions of the brand have up to 180 calories and 40 grams of sugar per serving.) Most of these "juice" drinks are really just water and high-fructose corn syrup. If you drink just one of these a day, cut it out—you'll lose 19 pounds this year!

STEP 3
>Choose Smoothies Over Juice

Annual weight loss: 14½ pounds

What could be healthier than this: Langers Pomegranate Blueberry Plus? It's 100 percent juice, says so right on the label. But the "Plus" is juice concentrate, which is so sweet that Langers packs 30 grams of sugar in each 8-ounce glass: That's the sugar equivalent of two—two!—Snicker's Ice

Cream Bars. Juices strip the fiber out of fruits and concentrate their sugars. Zero Belly Smoothies keep the fruit intact, so you get all the healthy stuff—without the blast of sugar.

STEP 4

>Drop the Bottled Iced Tea

Annual weight loss: 13½ pounds

You may think a bottle of iced tea is healthier than a soda, but you're only about half right. First, once a tea is made and sits on a supermarket shelf for, oh, an entire NFL season, the nutrients have spent enough time exposed to light and air that they begin to break down. The fact is, store-bought teas typically lose 20 percent of EGCG/catechin content during the bottling process, which is why brewing your own makes a lot more sense. Plus, who knows what else has worked its way into that bottle? Snapple's All Natural Green Tea packs 120 calories and 30 grams of sugar, while Ssips Green Tea with Honey & Ginseng is sweetened not so much with honey but with high-fructose corn syrup.

ZERO BELLY TIP:

ON A DIET?
AVOID DIET SODA.

Diet sodas can pack on pounds, too. "Artificial sweeteners affect our sense of satiety," says Isabel Smith, MS, RD, of Isabel Smith Nutrition. "Our bodies have evolutionarily developed to expect a large amount of calories when we take in something exceedingly sweet, and those artificial sweeteners are from 400 times to 8,000 times sweeter than sugar. It causes a couple things to happen: The muscles in your stomach relax so you can take in food, and hormones are released. With artificial sweeteners, your body says, 'Wait a minute, you told me you were going to give me all this high-calorie food.' It can actually send some people searching for more food, out of lack of satisfaction."

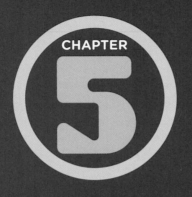

CHAPTER

5

FRUIT SMOOTHIES

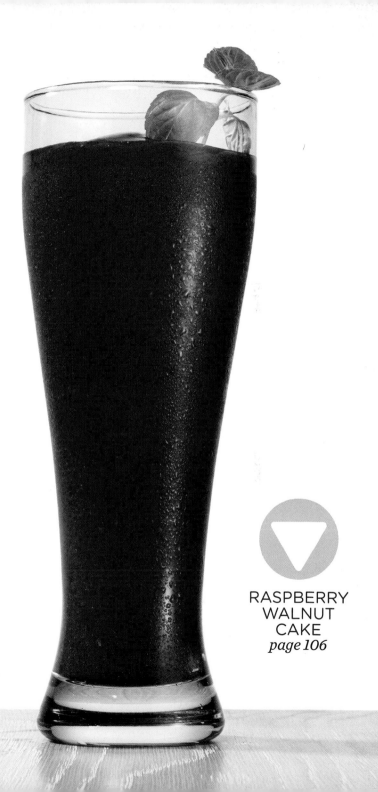

RASPBERRY
WALNUT
CAKE
page 106

Fruits are like people: They come in all sorts of shapes, sizes, colors, and styles, and each has its own temperament. Some are so sweet you can barely stand it, others so bitter you avoid them at all costs. But regardless of their individual qualities, all fruits have something to offer and deserve our utmost respect.

That said, my favorites are red fruits. While there are studies linking nearly every kind of fruit to some sort of health benefit, the most evidence tends to pile up around fruits that are red or reddish, like purple or orange fruits. For example, a study in the journal *Metabolism* found that eating half a red grapefruit before a meal may help reduce visceral fat and lower cholesterol levels. Another study found that tart cherries reduce belly fat; blueberries, strawberries, and raspberries have also been linked to lower abdominal fat accumulation.

So while a number of different fruits will show up in this collection, expect many of your smoothies from this chapter to have a cool red or purple hue. That's a sign that you're getting a massive hit of antioxidants and fat-fighting fiber.

All recipes make one serving.

APPLE PI

Pink Lady apples are among the most nutrient-rich varieties, according to a study at the University of Western Australia. This smoothie combines the apple with vanilla and cinnamon flavors to give you a uniquely autumnal fruit drink.

¼ **frozen banana**

½ **Pink Lady apple with peel,** seeded and quartered

½ **cup unsweetened almond milk**

1 teaspoon flaxseed oil

3.14 dashes of ground cinnamon

1 scoop vanilla plant-based protein powder

Water to blend (optional but recommended)

273 calories
7.4 g fat
27 g carbs
5.5 g fiber
15 g sugar
26 g protein

COCO-CARAMEL APPLE

A perfect Indian summer recipe: Nutmeg, one of the top Zero Belly spices, contains a compound called macelignan that helps protect cells from sun damage, according to a 2012 study in *Biological and Pharmaceutical Bulletin.* For a vitamin A boost, consider popping some pureed pumpkin into the mix!

1 Pink Lady apple with peel, cored and sliced

¼ cup unsweetened light coconut milk

¼ cup unsweetened almond milk

1 teaspoon pumpkin pie spice

1 teaspoon nutmeg

1 scoop plain plant-based protein powder

3 ice cubes

Water to blend (optional)

299 calories
16.9 g fat
12 g carbs
3.8 g fiber
5.5 g sugar
27 g protein

AVOCADO TART

The mellowness of the avocado and the tartness of the berries go together like guitar and bass. As blueberries tend to be high in pesticides, I stick strictly to organic blueberries.

½ cup frozen blueberries

½ cup unsweetened almond milk

¼ avocado

1 scoop vanilla plant-based protein powder

3 ice cubes

¼ cup water or more to blend

237 calories
6.7 g fat
19 g carbs
5.2 g fiber
10 g sugar
27 g protein

MANGO MUSCLE-UP

A classic from the original Zero Belly Diet, this pairs the sweetness of mango with muscle-building proteins.

⅔ **cup frozen mango chunks**

½ **tablespoon almond butter**

½ **cup unsweetened almond milk**

1 scoop plain plant-based protein powder

Water to blend (optional)

258 calories
6 g fat
19 g carbs
5 g fiber
15 g sugar
30 g protein

FRESH OFF THE OAT

Oatmeal is a secret smoothie booster that provides both protein and fiber, and helps to give your smoothie a thicker, creamier texture. The powder and banana will also thicken your drink, so add more almond milk if you need and make sure you're using a powerful blender.

¼ **cup frozen blueberries**

⅓ **frozen banana**

2 **tablespoons rolled oats**, cooked

2 **teaspoons almonds**

½ **cup unsweetened almond milk**

1 **scoop plain plant-based protein powder**
(hemp is recommended here)

Water to blend (optional but recommended)

271 calories
5.4 g fat
29 g carbs
5.4 g fiber
11 g sugar
29 g protein

STRAWBERRY PISTACHIO CREAM

Those Hulk-colored nuts have their own special fat-burning powers. In a recent study, one group was fed unsalted pistachios, while the other group was not. The pistachio group lost more belly chub.

½ cup frozen strawberries

¼ cup pistachios

½ avocado, peeled, pitted and quartered

3 ice cubes

1 teaspoon vanilla extract

1 scoop vanilla plant-based protein powder

Water to blend (necessary)

266 calories
9 g fat
18 g carbs
5 g fiber
8 g sugar
30 g protein

PIÑA COLADA

Resist the urge to add rum.
This vitamin-packed smoothie is one
of the lowest-calorie ways to get
your protein, fiber and healthy fats.

½ cup unsweetened light coconut milk

½ cup diced pineapple
(fresh, frozen, or canned in juice)

¼ frozen banana

2 fresh basil leaves

½ scoop plain plant-based protein powder

Water to blend (optional)

205 calories
7 g fat
21 g carbs
2 g fiber
11 g sugar
14 g protein

GINGER-BASIL GRAPEFRUIT

We don't often think of savory herbs like basil when it comes to smoothies, but its summery flavor is just the extra payoff for its cancer-fighting carotenoids. Here, I've used it to cut the tang of the grapefruit and ginger. This is more like a juice than a smoothie—in a good way.

½ **grapefruit, peeled**, with bitter insides removed (in other words, just the segments)

½ **frozen banana**

½ **cup unsweetened almond milk**

½ **teaspoon fresh ginger,** peeled and chopped

1 sprig fresh basil

2 ice cubes

½ **scoop plain plant-based protein powder** (try hemp)

Water to blend (optional)

231 calories
28 g fat
26 g carbs
4.4 g fiber
14 g sugar
27 g protein

PEACH DREAM

Peaches, nectarines and other stone fruits are high in phenolic compounds that help ward off belly fat, high cholesterol, and insulin resistance. Because they're low in sugar, I like to combine them with other fruits, like strawberries, to give a smoothie a fully rounded flavor.

½ **peach**

2 strawberries

¼ **avocado,** peeled, pitted, and quartered

½ **cup unsweetened almond milk**

3 ice cubes

½ **scoop vanilla plant-based protein powder**

Water to blend (optional)

214 calories
11.7 g fat
11.8 g carbs
5.1 g fiber
5.5 g sugar
15.1 g protein

BLUEBERRY DAZZLER

Consider using wild blueberries (you can find them in the freezer section); they're higher in just about every nutrient than conventional blueberries.

½ cup frozen blueberries

½ tablespoon almond butter

½ cup unsweetened almond milk

1 scoop vanilla plant-based protein powder

Water to blend (necessary here)

254 calories
7 g fat
19 g carbs
4 g fiber
10 g sugar
20 g protein

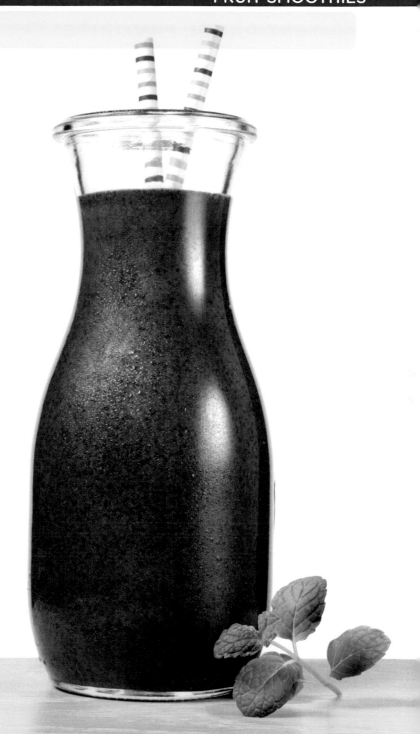

"PEACH OUT" PEACH OAT COBBLER

Like a light, summery bowl of oats—this is comfort food in a glass. Unless it's August and the peaches in your neck of the woods are perfect, opt for frozen peaches instead. The vanilla in the protein powder will combine with the peaches for a bright, warm, and hearty drink.

½ **peach**

½ **frozen banana**

2 tablespoons rolled oats

½ **cup unsweetened almond milk**

1 teaspoon ground flaxseed

1 scoop vanilla plant-based protein powder

Water to blend (optional)

277 calories
4 g fat
33 g carbs
6 g fiber
14 g sugar
28 g protein

STRAWBERRY BANANA

Almond butter is one of the best possible sources of vitamin E, and in this drink it provides a nice nutty note to the fruity flavors of banana and strawberry.

⅓ **cup frozen strawberries**

¼ **frozen banana**

½ **tablespoon almond butter**

½ **cup unsweetened almond milk**

½ **scoop vanilla plant-based protein powder**

Water to blend (optional)

232 calories
5 g fat
16 g carbs
4 g fiber
8 g sugar
29 g protein

GREEN RASPBERRY

One of the great tricks of these smoothies is that you can sneak a relatively neutral vegetable like spinach into almost any of them. Spinach is one of the best sources of folate, which has been shown to reduce the risk of everything from diabetes to dementia.

⅓ cup raspberries

½ frozen banana

1 cup fresh spinach

1 teaspoon flaxseed oil

½ cup unsweetened almond milk

1 scoop plain plant-based protein powder

3 ice cubes

Water to blend (optional)

286 calories
8 g fat
27 g carbs
7 g fiber
12 g sugar
29 g protein

THE STRAW VOCADO

It may not look, act or taste like it, but the avocado is a fruit (so are olives). When you add avocado to a smoothie you give it a big boost of belly-satisfying monounsaturated fats. Note: Avocado will dramatically reduce your appetite for up to four hours. Deploy accordingly.

¼ **avocado,** peeled, pitted, and quartered

½ **cup frozen strawberries**

½ **cup unsweetened almond milk**

1 scoop plain or vanilla plant-based protein powder

Squeeze of fresh lemon juice

2 ice cubes

Water to blend (optional)

289 calories
12 g fat
18 g carbs
7 g fiber
8 g sugar
28 g protein

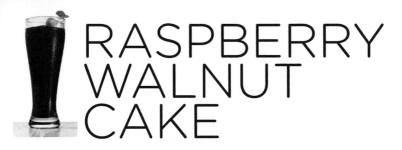

RASPBERRY WALNUT CAKE

No fruit carries the fiber punch of raspberries. They grow wild along the driveway of my house in Long Island, and friends' children will often collect a big bucket in early July. Otherwise, I opt for the frozen variety, which are nutritionally superior to most of what you'll find in the produce section of your supermarket.

⅓ cup frozen raspberries

½ frozen banana

1 tablespoon walnuts

1 tablespoon walnuts

½ cup unsweetened almond milk

Water to blend (optional but recommended here)

For topping: **1 piece of dark chocolate,** grated

285 calories
7 g fat
26 g carbs
7 g fiber
12 g sugar
30 g protein

 After blending, grate dark chocolate on top of smoothie and serve.

GINGER MAN

Ginger packs high levels of health-boosting phytonutrients. But use fresh ginger: Chances are you bought that powdered ginger in your cabinet three years ago when you made a pumpkin pie, and it's been losing potency ever since. To keep fresh ginger on hand, break it into small chunks and freeze it, then allow to defrost before grating.

½ cup frozen strawberries

¼ frozen banana

1 cup unsweetened almond milk

1 tablespoon fresh ginger, peeled and chopped

1 teaspoon ground flaxseed

Dash of ground pepper

1 scoop plain plant-based protein powder

Water to blend (optional)

264 calories
5 g fat
26 g carbs
6 g fiber
11 g sugar
29 g protein

GREAT GRAPE

This might be the most nutritious drink you'll ever savor. Resveratrol, the nutrient found in highest levels in the skins of red grapes, acts directly on the epigenetic mechanisms that control weight gain in general and belly fat in particular. Anda recent study at William Paterson University found that watercress has the highest

½ cup frozen seedless red grapes

¼ frozen banana

1 tablespoon ground flaxseed

1 cup watercress

5 fresh mint leaves

½ cup unsweetened almond milk

½ scoop plain plant-based protein powder

3 ice cubes

Water to blend (optional)

279 calories
5.5 g fat
28 g carbs
9.2 g fiber
14 g sugar
30 g protein

MELON BALLER

Two of summer's superfoods combine powers in this extremely light recipe. Serve it wth a fresh sprig of basil or mint. You can also whip up a version with just the melon, watercress, and ice for a low-calorie refresher that's perfect for when you finish mowing the lawn.

1 cup frozen watermelon,
  seedless, with rind removed

1 cups watercress

½ cup unsweetened almond milk

1 scoop vanilla plant-based protein powder

198 calories
2 g fat
17.8 g carbs
1.3 g fiber
12.5 g sugar
27.6 g protein

DETOX WATERMELON

A study at the University of Kentucky found that watermelon may improve lipid profiles and lower fat accumulation, while another study found that the melon helped reduce post-exercise muscle soreness.

1 cup watermelon, seedless, with rind removed

3 shavings fresh ginger

½ cup unsweetened almond milk

⅛ teaspoon cayenne pepper

4 ice cubes

1 scoop plain plant-based protein powder

TEST PANEL FAVORITE!

BANANA SPLIT

Valentine's Day in a glass. Don't under-estimate the healing powers of dark chocolate—it's not there as a gimmick. When you combine fruit and dark chocolate (at least 70 percent cacao), you accelerate the release of butyrate, a compound made in your large intestine that tells your fat-storage genes to chill out.

1 frozen banana

4 fresh cherries, pitted

2 dark chocolate squares

1 teaspoon vanilla extract

½ cup unsweetened almond milk

1 scoop vanilla plant-based protein powder

2 ice cubes

Topping: 1 more cherry

280 calories
3 g fat
35 g carbs
6 g fiber
17 g sugar
28 g protein

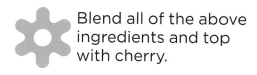 Blend all of the above ingredients and top with cherry.

CHERRIES 'N' CREAM

"Tastes like birthday cake" is what I hear when I serve this to guests. Despite its 28 grams of protein, this smoothie is light and perfect for springtime.

1 frozen banana

5 fresh cherries, pitted

½ cup unsweetened almond milk

1 scoop vanilla plant-based protein powder

268 calories
3 g fat
34 g carbs
5 g fiber
17 g sugar
28 g protein

FRESH BLUEBERRY

This beauty from *Zero Belly Cookbook* combines the antioxidants of blueberries with muscle-building almond butter.

½ cup frozen blueberries

1½ teaspoon almond butter,
    no-salt-added

½ cup unsweetened almond milk

1 scoop vanilla plant-based protein powder

Water to blend (optional)

232 calories
6 g fat
16 g carbs
3 g fiber
9 g sugar
28 g protein

6

GREEN
SMOOTHIES

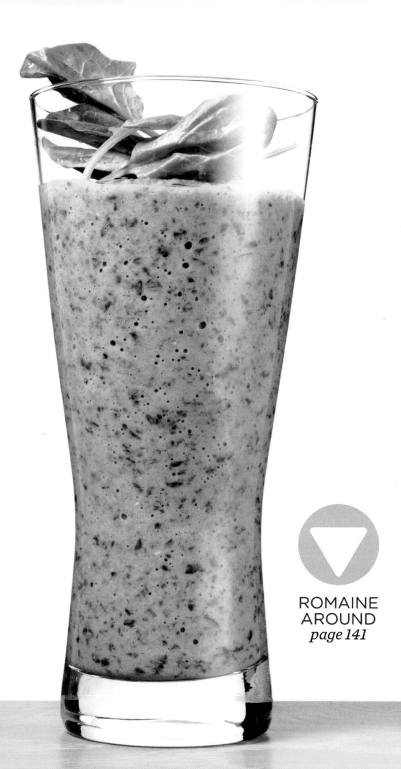

ROMAINE
AROUND
page 141

When you think of green drinks, you probably think first about green juices. Juicing has been an insanely hot nutritional trend ever since Beyoncé claimed to use the Master Cleanse to get ready for *Dreamgirls*.

Popping into a juice bar for a cold cup of extruded kale juice may be all the rage, but when it comes to both nutritional impact and weight-loss power, juices can't hold a candle to smoothies. First, most commercial juices use apple juice, which is a high-sugar, low-nutrient base. (Most of the nutritional impact of an apple is in its skin, not the white pulp where most of the juice is extracted from.) Second, juicing strips all the natural fiber out of produce, which is like stripping the political backstabbing out of *House of Cards*: The rough stuff is what makes it good. And third, juices lack fat and protein; without these crucial elements, you're getting no fat-burning, metabolism-boosting benefits.

Next time you want to drink your veggies, blend up one of these seriously nutritious recipes.

All recipes make one serving.

KALE TO THE CHIEF

In addition to sweetening this recipe, the mango delivers three-fourths of your daily vitamin C requirement. And kale is a rich source of the nutrient sulforaphane, which controls the genes that determine whether a stem cell turns into a fat cell.

1 cup kale

½ cup mango, peeled and pitted

¼ avocado, peeled, pitted, and quartered

6 fresh mint leaves

1 tablespoon fresh lemon juice

1 cup coconut water

1 scoop plain plant-based protein powder

Water to blend (optional)

301 calories
12 g fat
19 g carbs
6.5 g fiber
3.4 g sugar
30 g protein

SPRIG OF PARSLEY

This is the world's most overlooked superfood: Studies show that parsley is actually more dense with nutrients than kale, dandelion greens, or romaine lettuce. Combine it with superheroes like watercress and chia and you've got a mighty fat-fighting drink.

¼ cup fresh parsley (include the stems)

½ cup watercress

½ cup frozen strawberries

½ frozen banana

1 teaspoon chia seeds

1 scoop plain plant-based protein powder

Water to blend (optional)

214 calories
2 g fat
22 g carbs
4 g fiber
10 g sugar
28.5 g protein

ON THE WATERCRESS

Watercress is not only the No. 1 most powerful vegetable known to man, according to a recent study, but its nutritional calling card is folate. A study in the *British Journal of Nutrition* found that those with the highest folate levels lose 8.5 times more weight when dieting than those with the lowest.

1 cup watercress

¼ apple with peel, seeded and quartered

¼ avocado, peeled, pitted, and quartered

½ cup water

½ cup unsweetened almond milk

1 scoop plain plant-based protein powder

3 ice cubes

Water to blend (optional)

295 calories
12 g fat
18 g carbs
7 g fiber
7 g sugar
29 g protein

GREEN MONSTER

This filling, creamy drink isn't what you think of when you imagine a classic green drink: It's a lot more like a milk shake than a juice. But it will affect you in the exact opposite way: A 2012 study in *The American Journal of Clinical Nutrition* found that consuming pears (as well as apples and blueberries) reduced the risk of diabetes.

½ **Bosc pear,** seeded and quartered

½ **frozen banana**

¼ **avocado,** peeled, pitted, and quartered

½ **cup baby spinach,** loosely packed

½ **cup no-sugar-added apple juice**

¼ **cup water**

1 scoop plain plant-based protein powder

3 ice cubes

Water to blend (optional)

271 calories
6 g fat
40 g carbs
8 g fiber
18 g sugar
15 g protein

UNDER THE COLLARD

If you're vegan, collard greens should be high on your list of must-eat foods. They're far and away the best vegetable source of choline, a nutrient (mostly found in egg yolks and meat) that turns off the genes for abdominal weight gain.

1 cup collard greens, stemmed and chopped

2 tablespoons fresh lime juice

1 cup unsweetened almond milk

1 scoop plain plant-based protein powder

3 ice cubes

Water to blend (optional)

237 calories
9 g fat
11 g carbs
4 g fiber
3 g sugar
28 g protein

LEMON KALE PROTEIN DETOX

Putting lemon in your blender is like taking out a nutrition insurance policy for your smoothie. That's because a significant percentage of the antioxidant polyphenols in any food or drink break down before they reach your bloodstream. But researchers at Purdue University discovered that adding lemon juice to the equation helped preserve the polyphenols.

½ **lemon,** peeled and seeded

½ **frozen banana**

1 cup kale

½ **cup unsweetened almond milk**

1 scoop plain plant-based protein powder

3 ice cubes

Water to blend (optional)

254 calories
7 g fat
20 g carbs
5 g fiber
10 g sugar
30 g protein

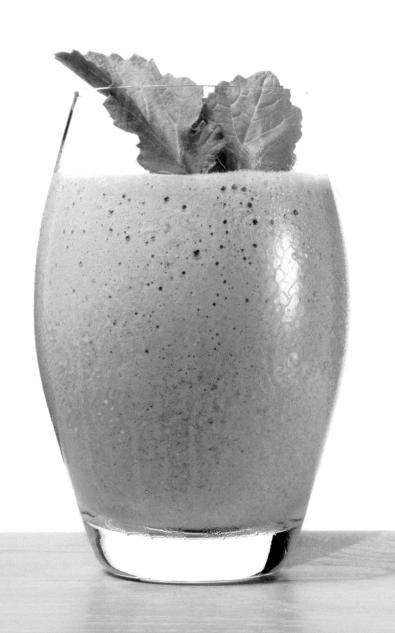

CHICORY ROOT BEER

Add chicory to the list of overlooked fat-fighters. More nutritious than lettuce or even kale, chicory is the primary source of inulin, the soluble fiber that's added to products like Activia to promote a healthy belly biome.

½ **cup chicory**

½ **cup spinach**

¼ **apple with peel,** seeded and quartered

½ **frozen banana**

1 tsp chia seeds

1 cup water

1 scoop plain plant-based protein powder

Touch of honey

Water to blend (optional)

After blending, add a splash of soda water for fizz.

231 calories
2 g fat
27 g carbs
5.5 g fiber
14 g sugar
28 g protein

THE CUKE-CLEAR OPTION

Cucumber and watercress keep the flavor mellow, but it's kiwi—one of the best plant sources of omega-3 fatty acids—that steals the show here.

½ **cucumber,** peeled and seeded

½ **kiwi,** peeled

1 cup watercress

½ cup unsweetened almond milk

1 scoop plain plant-based protein powder

4 ice cubes

Water to blend (optional)

214 calories
3 g fat
18 g carbs
4.5 g fiber
8 g sugar
19 g protein

HEMP CAT

Combining hemp and chia seeds gives you a superdose of omega-3 fatty acids. And hemp seeds, by weight, provide more protein than even beef or fish.

¾ **cup baby kale**

½ **frozen banana**

1 teaspoon hemp seeds

½ **tablespoon chia seeds**

½ **cup unsweetened almond milk**

1 scoop vanilla plant-based protein powder

Water to blend (optional)

270 calories
6 g fat
26 g carbs
6 g fiber
10 g sugar
29 g protein

MEET YOUR MATCHA

A superhealthy version of the Shamrock Shake: One study found men who drank green tea containing 136 milligrams EGCG—what you'll find in a single 4-gram serving of matcha—lost twice as much weight than a placebo group, and four times as much visceral (belly) fat over the course of three months. And the menthol in mint has been shown to help ease digestion.

1 cup spinach, loosely packed

1 tablespoon matcha green tea powder

¼ avocado, peeled, pitted, and quartered

4 fresh mint leaves

½ cup unsweetened almond milk

1 scoop vanilla plant-based protein powder

Water to blend (optional)

290 calories
12 g fat
16 g carbs
9 g fiber
3 g sugar
30 g protein

GREEN MATCHA TEA

Matcha is the powdered tea used in Japanese tea ceremonies. Some studies have shown the concentration of metabolism-boosting EGCG in matcha to be as much as 137 times greater than the amount you'll find in most store-bought green tea. EGCG can simultaneously boost lipolysis (the breakdown of fat) and block adipogenesis (the formation of fat cells) particularly in the belly.

½ **cup baby spinach,** loosely packed
½ **frozen banana**
1 teaspoon matcha green tea powder
1 teaspoon ground cinnamon
1 scoop vanilla plant-based protein powder
Water to blend (optional)

226 calories
1.3 g fat
26 g carbs
6 g fiber
13 g sugar
28 g protein

TEA FOR ONE

I can't recommend green tea enough as a smoothie enhancer. In fact, people who drink green tea regularly have nearly 20 percent less body fat than those who don't, according to one 10-year Taiwanese study. And EGCG, the unique ingredient in green tea, can deactivate the genetic triggers for diabetes and obesity.

1 cup green tea

½ frozen banana

2 tablespoons fresh lemon juice

⅛ avocado

1 scoop vanilla plant-based protein powder

Water to blend (optional)

245 calories
6 g fat
23 g carbs
5 g fiber
11 g sugar
26 g protein

BANANA SALAD

There are times when you crave something that isn't fruity or sweet, and this recipe is the perfect solution. A true folate festival, thanks to the kale and spinach, it really is like a salad in a cup—except much easier to eat when you're driving to work.

1 cup spinach

½ cup kale

½ frozen banana

½ cup unsweetened almond milk

1 scoop plain plant-based protein powder

Splash of red wine vinegar

Water to blend (optional)

237 calories
3 g fat
25 g carbs
5 g fiber
10 g sugar
29 g protein

BEET GREEN

Save the beets for another smoothie; for this one, all you need are the greens.

1 cup beet greens, washed

½ cup frozen strawberries

1 teaspoon coconut oil

1 cup unsweetened almond milk

1 scoop plain plant-based protein powder

247 calories
9 g fat
16 g carbs
5.5 g fiber
7 g sugar
27 g protein

LEAF RELIEF

Some of my favorite restaurants offer a blackberry-and-spinach salad, so I was inspired to blend them up along with a squeeze of lemon. Glad I did.

½ cup frozen blackberries

½ lemon

1 cup spinach

1 cup unsweetened almond milk

1 scoop plain or flavored plant-based protein powder

219 calories
4.7 g fat
18.5 g carbs
8 g fiber
7 g sugar
28 g protein

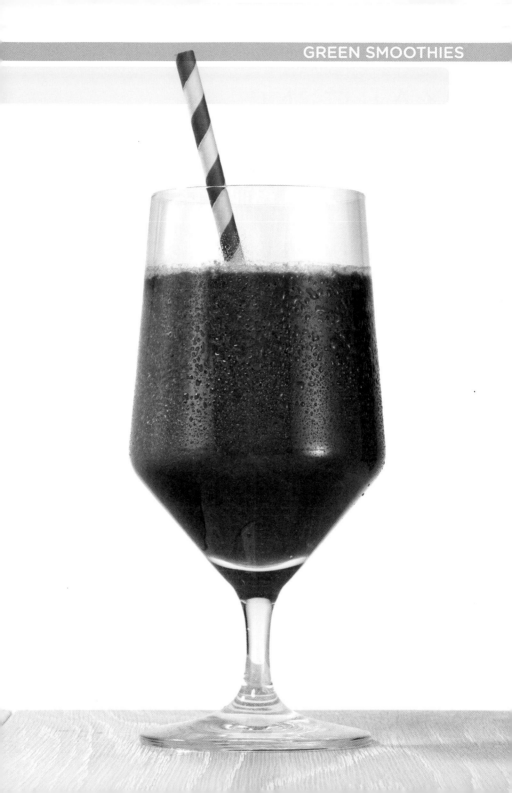

KALE 'N' HEARTY

Want to keep your belly biome happy? To make sure your gut is in good shape, you need to feed your abdominal allies something called fructooligosaccharides, or FOS, a type of fiber found in fruits and leafy greens. This drink will get the party started and help heal your gut while enticing your taste buds.

1 cup kale

cup chopped cucumber, peeled and seeded

pear, seeded and quartered

Squeeze of fresh lime juice

1 scoop plain or vanilla plant-based protein powder

cup water

2 ice cubes

217 calories
1 g fat
26 g carbs
5 g fiber
11 g sugar
28 g protein

TEST PANEL FAVORITE!

COCO-NUTS

You may think you're doing yourself a favor by eschewing peanuts for more exotic nut spreads, but there's absolutely nothing wrong with standing by plain old peanut butter. It's higher in protein than any other nut (nearly four times as much protein as cashews) and packed with folate as well. Plus, it's the perfect foil for coconut.

½ cup unsweetened light coconut milk

1 cup kale

½ frozen banana

1 tablespoon unsalted peanut butter

½ scoop vanilla plant-based protein powder

½ cup ice

273 calories
11 g fat
28 g carbs
5 g fiber
9 g sugar
19 g protein

ROLLING
IN GREEN

This green monster combines two of my favorite leafy greens—spinach and watercress—with some green veggies and an avocado. Your neighbors will be green with envy.

1 cup spinach

1 cup watercress

¼ avocado

¼ cucumber

¼ cup celery, diced

squeeze of lime

1 scoop plain plant-based protein powder

Water to blend (¾ to 1 cup)

266 calories
10 g fat
15 g carbs
7 g fiber
5 g sugar
28 g protein

GREENER PASTURES

Why oats in your smoothie? A Tufts University study found that participants who ate three or more servings of whole grains (like oats) had 10 percent less belly fat than people who ate the same amount of calories from refined carbs. The more of these little disks of dietary dynamite you eat (or drink), the better.

½ **frozen banana**

½ **cup unsweetened almond milk**

1 **cup spinach**

¼ **cup rolled oats**

1 **scoop chocolate plant-based protein powder**

Water to blend (optional)

284 calories
4 g fat
35 g carbs
6 g fiber
11 g sugar
30 g protein

ORANGESICLE

Orange juice, no. Oranges, yes! In addition to getting the orange's natural fiber, you're also getting a youth makeover: A study in *Evolution and Human Behavior* found that people who ate more oranges had a more sun-kissed complexion than those who didn't consume as much, thanks to nutrients called carotenoids.

½ **orange,** peeled and seeded

½ **frozen banana**

1 cup spinach, tightly packed

½ **cup unsweetened almond milk**

1 teaspoon flaxseed oil

1 scoop vanilla plant-based protein powder

3 ice cubes

Water to blend (optional)

295 calories
7 g fat
32 g carbs
6 g fiber
19 g sugar
28 g protein

ALMOND SALAD

Perhaps the absolute best source of vitamin E, almond butter blends perfectly with vanilla and banana to create a subtle, nutty flavor—you'll never even know that spinach crashed this party.

1 cup spinach

1 tablespoon almond butter

½ frozen banana

½ cup unsweetened almond milk

¾ cup water

1 scoop vanilla plant-based protein powder

294 calories
10 g fat
24 g carbs
6 g fiber
11 g sugar
31 g protein

THE CHARD

It's not as fun a name to drop as, say, "broccolini," but chard might be your best defense against diabetes. Recent research has shown that these powerhouse leaves contain at least 13 different polyphenol antioxidants, including anthocyanins–anti-inflammatory compounds that could offer protection from type 2 diabetes. Researchers from the University of East Anglia analyzed questionnaires and blood samples of about 2,000 people and found that those with the highest dietary intakes of anthocyanins had lower insulin resistance and better blood glucose regulation.

1 cup chard

½ frozen banana

1 teaspoon coconut oil

1 inch fresh ginger

1 cup unsweetened almond milk

1 scoop plain plant-based protein powder

290 calories
9 g fat
26 g carbs
5 g fiber
10 g sugar
28 g protein

TEST PANEL FAVORITE!

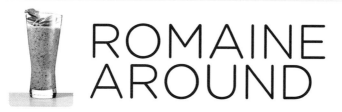

ROMAINE AROUND

We think of romaine lettuce as the crispy stuff at the bottom of a Caesar salad, but it's one of the 10 most nutritious vegetables around, and higher in fiber than almost any other form of lettuce. And because it's mostly water, it makes this smoothie a real thirst-quencher.

1 cup romaine lettuce

½ cup spinach

½ apple with peel, seeded and quartered

1 tablespoon chia seeds

½ cup unsweetened almond milk

1 scoop plain plant-based protein powder

Water to blend (optional)

280 calories
5.8 g fat
27 g carbs
10 g fiber
12 g sugar
201 g protein

THE BLUEGRASS FESTIVAL

Blueberries, spinach, and avocado all in one dish: It's like an *Avengers* movie. The fat in the avocados helps make the folate in the spinach more bioavailable: Studies show that women who eat foods with high water content, such as spinach, have lower BMIs and smaller waistlines than those who don't.

¼ cup blueberries

1 cup spinach, chopped

¼ avocado, peeled, pitted, and quartered

½ cup unsweetened almond milk

1 scoop plain plant-based protein powder

Water to blend (recommended)

292 calories
12 g fat
18 g carbs
7 g fiber
7 g sugar
29 g carbs

ZERO BELLY TIP:

SAY BOO TO BOOZE!

A study published in the *American Journal of Nutrition* showed that alcohol is one of the biggest drivers of excess food intake. Another study published in the journal *Obesity* has suggested that this may be because alcohol heightens our senses. Researchers found that women who'd received the equivalent of about two drinks in the form of an alcohol infusion ate 30 percent more food than those who'd received a saline solution.

7

NUTTY & CHOCOLATY SMOOTHIES

—

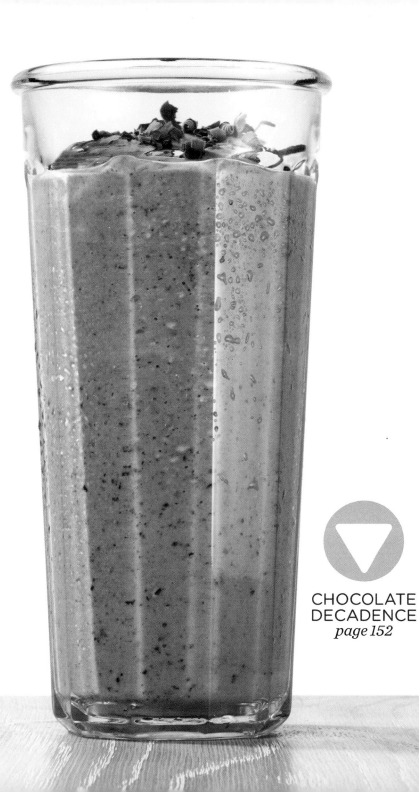

CHOCOLATE
DECADENCE
page 152

Have you ever heard of the "health halo"? It's a term nutrition experts use to describe foods that use a healthy-sounding word like *natural* on their labels, or add ingredients that people think of as good for you ("Now with chia!"), but which are really junk at heart.

This chapter is the reverse of that theory. These drinks are tremendously nutritious—packed with as much, or more, fiber, protein, and healthy fats as any other drinks in the whole book. But they seem like they're bad for you. How can drinks that seem like they came right from the ice cream shop flatten your belly so effectively?

These are the drinks you'll whip up on a night when you want something to satisfy your ice cream jones. They're the recipes you'll lean on when your kids are complaining that they want something sweet for dessert. And they're the drinks you'll use to reward yourself after a hard day at work or in the gym. Deep, comforting, and delicious, these filling smoothies taste more like dessert than what they really are—powerful weight-loss weapons.

All recipes make one serving.

TEST PANEL FAVORITE!

DARK CHOCOLATE BANANA NUT

Four words that combine to sound like a jam session at Ben & Jerry's house. The density of the banana will have you convinced you're drinking a milkshake, while the omega-3s in the walnuts will keep your mind sharp and your belly lean.

½ banana

1 teaspoon dark chocolate morsels (dairy free)

1 cup unsweetened almond milk

⅛ cup chopped walnuts

6 ice cubes

⅓ cup chocolate plant-based protein powder

Water to blend (optional)

229 calories
11 g fat
26 g carbs
7 g fiber
10 g sugar
28 g protein

ALMOND JOY

Mixing fruit and chocolate together is a trick that turbocharges your fat-melting mechanism. Fruit is fermented at the bottom of your digestive system, where it releases the appetite anti-inflammatory compound butyrate; cocoa helps accelerate that process.

¼ cup blueberries

1 tablespoon unsweetened cocoa powder

2 tablespoons shredded coconut

1 cup unsweetened almond milk

¼ cup black beans

6 ice cubes

¼ cup chocolate plant-based protein powder

Water to blend (optional)

294 calories
11 g fat
24 g carbs
10 g fiber
7 g sugar
25 g protein

CHERRY CHOCOLATE TART

Cherries and banana don't spend nearly as much time together as they ought to, and you'll agree after you taste this. Using an entire banana gives you an extra hit of resistant starch, a type of carbohydrate that resists digestion.

½ cup cherries, pitted

½ banana

1 tablespoon unsweetened cocoa powder

½ cup unsweetened almond milk

Dash of nutmeg

¼ cup black beans

6 ice cubes

¼ cup chocolate plant-based protein powder

Water to blend (optional)

294 calories
2 g fat
41 g carbs
11 g fiber
14 g sugar
25 g protein

THE PEANUT BUTTER CUP

Like a Reese's, but without the bad carbs!
A classic from the original *Zero Belly Diet*.

½ **frozen banana**

½ **tablespoon peanut butter**

1 **tablespoon unsweetened cocoa powder**

½ **cup unsweetened almond milk**

1 **scoop chocolate plant-based protein powder**

258 calories
6 g fat
20 g carbs
5 g fiber
14 g sugar
30 g protein

VALENTINE'S DAY

Strawberries can get overwhelmed by peanut butter, but the more delicate flavor of cashews helps them stand out in this recipe. And cashews are particularly rich in proanthocyanidins, a class of flavanols that help boost the immune system. You won't even notice the black beans.

1 cup frozen strawberries

1 tablespoon cashew butter

⅓ cup unsweetened almond milk

¼ cup black beans

¼ cup chocolate plant-based protein powder

2 ice cubes

300 calories
9 g fat
30 g carbs
9 g fiber
9 g sugar
26 g protein

Blend all ingredients until smooth, and then shave a square of dark chocolate on top for presentation.

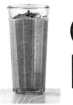

CHOCOLATE DECADENCE

This recipe is adapted from one of our favorites from *Zero Belly Cookbook*. We loved it so much we had to include it here as well. For 150-plus recipes that melt belly fat first—featuring foods you love— check out the cookbook today.

½ banana

¼ ripe avocado, peeled, pitted, and quartered

¼ cup black beans

½ cup unsweetened almond milk

¼ cup chocolate plant-based protein powder

6 ice cubes

Water to blend (optional)

300 calories
9 g fat
34 g carb
11 g fiber
9 g sugar
25 g protein

CHOCO-COLADA

Coconut is a super-trendy food, and for good reason: The fat in coconut is particularly high in lauric acid, a type of fat that's more difficult for the body to convert into body fat than other types of dietary fat; as a result, your body tends to burn it for energy.

2 teaspoons ground flaxseed

1 tablespoon shredded coconut

1 cup unsweetened almond milk

½ cup crushed pineapple

⅓ cup chocolate plant-based protein powder

6 ice cubes

Water to blend (optional)

296 calories
9 g fat
28 g carbs
6 g fiber
9 g sugar
27 g protein

PEACHY KEEN

As fruits go, bananas and peaches are polar opposites: bananas provide fiber and a rich consistency, while peaches add antioxidants for very few calories.

1 cup frozen peaches

½ banana

1 cup unsweetened almond milk

1 teaspoon vanilla extract

⅓ cup vanilla plant-based protein powder

½ cup ice cubes

Water to blend (optional)

287 calories
3 g fat
36 g carbs
5 g fiber
22 g sugar
29 g protein

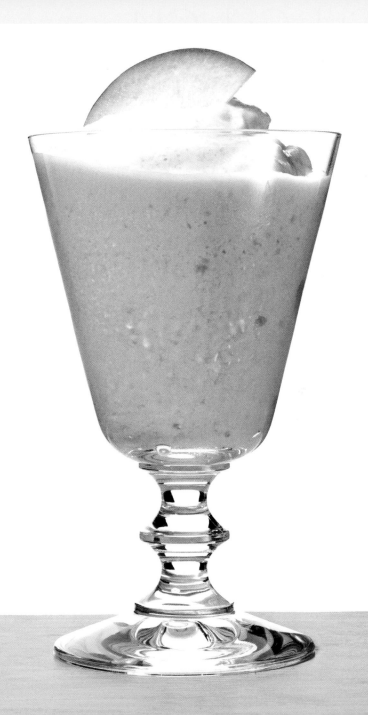

CH-CH-CH-CHOCOLATE CHIA

The fiber in the chia seeds adds an extra level of fat-burning fun to a drink that tastes like a dessert.

½ banana

1 kiwi

2 teaspoons ground chia seeds

¼ cup black beans

½ cup unsweetened almond milk

¼ cup chocolate plant-based protein powder

3 ice cubes

Water to blend (optional)

298 calories
4 g fat
43 g carbs
14 g fiber
15 g sugar
26 g protein

FLAXING & RELAXING

Flax oil is the single most potent source of omega-3 fatty acids; the ½ tablespoon in this recipe will give you 3,600 milligrams of the stuff, about twice what you'll get from a 3-ounce portion of salmon. And omega-3s are shown to help reduce stress, so you really will be "flaxing and relaxing."

¼ **cup pomegranate seeds**

½ **cup frozen blueberries**

½ **tablespoon flaxseed oil**

½ **cup unsweetened almond milk**

⅓ **cup scoop chocolate plant-based protein powder**

3 ice cubes

Water to blend (optional)

288 calories
10 g fat
25 g carbs
7 g fiber
14 g sugar
27 g protein

CA-CAO POW!

This drink packs a tremendous protein punch, not just from the vanilla powder but from the cacao (which delivers a gram per teaspoon) and the spirulina, a type of algae that's about 60 percent protein. Like quinoa, it's a complete protein, meaning it can be converted directly into muscle in the body.

1 cup spinach

½ cup blueberries

½ teaspoon spirulina

1 tablespoon cacao powder

1 tablespoon ground chia seeds

½ cup unsweetened almond milk

¼ cup vanilla plant-based protein powder

Water to blend (optional)

255 calories
5 g fat
27 g carb
11 g fiber
8 g sugar
28 g protein

IT'S A DATE

You'll love this super sweet treat. Dates are higher in fructose than any other food, which explains why this drink tastes as if we added sugar to it. But that's natural fructose that comes with a shielding of fiber, so it won't spike your blood sugar. Watch tennis champ Novak Djokovic in the middle of a tournament—he eats dates in between sets to keep his energy up.

2 tablespoon almonds, blanched

1 tablespoon ground chia seeds

¼ teaspoon nutmeg

¼ teaspoon cinnamon

1 date

1 cup unsweetened almond milk

1 cup ice

¼ cup vanilla plant-based protein powder

Water to blend (optional)

272 calories
12 g fat
18 g carb
5 g fiber
7 g sugar
25 g protein

VANILLA CHAI

Swap this in for your usual
A.M. Starbucks order.

½ **cup chai tea** (brewed from a tea bag and chilled)

½ **frozen banana**

½ **teaspoon ground cinnamon**

1½ **teaspoon almond butter,** no-salt-added

¼ **cup unsweetened almond milk**

½ **scoop vanilla plant-based protein powder**

Water to blend (optional)

219 calories
9 g fat
20 g carbs
4 g fiber
16 g sugar
17 g protein

VELVETY ELVIS

Okay, we took Elvis's favorite sandwich and turned it into a smoothie, but we added the super protein punch of spirulina. A tablespoon delivers 8 grams of metabolism-boosting protein for just 43 calories, plus half a day's allotment of vitamin B12.

½ frozen banana

1 tablespoon almond butter

1 tablespoon powdered spirulina

½ cup unsweetened almond milk

¼ cup plain plant-based protein powder

Water to blend (optional)

288 calories
10 g fat
25 g carb
5 g fiber
7 g sugar
30 g protein

CHOCOLATE BEAN

Beans? In a smoothie? Use canned or precooked beans for a thick, earthy protein and fiber punch. One study found that people who ate ¾ cup of beans daily weighed 6.6 pounds less, on average, than those who didn't, even though the bean eaters took in more calories.

½ **frozen banana**

¼ **cup black beans**

1 tsp nutmeg

1 cup unsweetened almond milk

⅓ **cup plant-based chocolate protein powder**

Water to blend (optional)

280 calories
3 g fat
31 g carbs
7 g fiber
9 g sugar
31 g protein

PEANUT BUTTER SANDWICH

One of my favorite food tricks is to make peanut butter & jelly sandwiches for kids, but to swap out the jelly for fresh berries (blackberries work best). The kids can never tell. You'll get the same nutritional upgrade from this smoothie recipe.

5 raspberries

5 blueberries

3 strawberries

1 tablespoon peanut butter, unsalted

½ cup unsweetened almond milk

¼ cup vanilla plant-based protein powder

½ cup ice cubes

Water to blend (optional)

255 calories
12 g fat
14 g carb
4 g fiber
9 g sugar
25 g protein

AVOCADO BLUES

You won't feel blue after drinking this, and you won't feel hungry, either: A study in *Nutrition Journal* found that participants who ate avocado for lunch reported a 40 percent decreased desire to eat for hours afterward. Blueberries and flaxseed add an extra nutritional boost.

¼ **avocado,** peeled, pitted, and quartered

½ **cup blueberries**

¼ **cup black beans**

1 tsp ground flaxseed

½ **cup unsweetened almond milk**

¼ **cup chocolate plant-based protein powder**

3 ice cubes

Water to blend (optional)

297 calories
10 g fat
30 g carbs
15 g fiber
9 g sugar
25 g protein

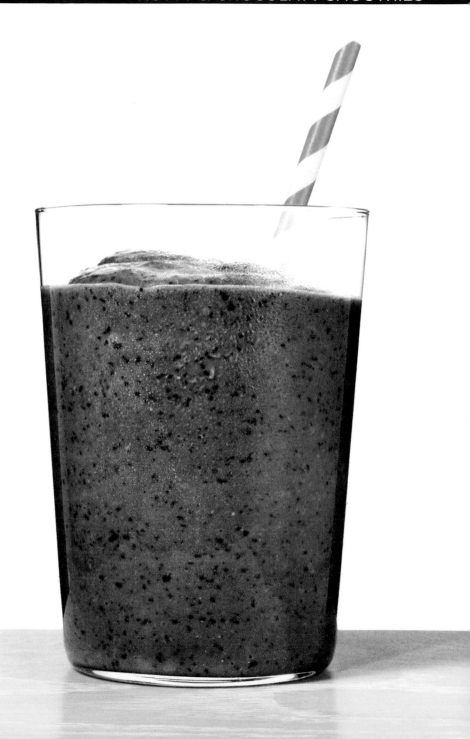

CANTALOUPE KICK

A great combination of flavors inspired by Mexican cuisine. Just ½ teaspoon of hot pepper can help reduce appetite after a meal, according to a study at Purdue University. And daily consumption of capsaicin, the active ingredient in cayenne, speeds abdominal weight loss, according to a study in the *American Journal of Clinical Nutrition*.

1 cup cantaloupe

½ cup mango

1 dash cayenne pepper

1 cup unsweetened almond milk

1 tablespoon ground chia seeds

⅓ cup chocolate plant-based protein powder

6 ice cubes

Water to blend (optional)

298 calories
5 g fat
35 g carbs
6 g fiber
23 g sugar
29 g protein

KEEP IT SIMPLE

This one really does keep it simple. In the end, all you need for a great smoothie is fiber, fat and protein, plus one plant or fruit source. The almond butter provides the first three, while the mix of chocolate and banana takes this flavor profile over the edge.

½ cup peaches

1 tablespoon almond butter

1 cup unsweetened almond milk

⅓ cup chocolate plant-based protein powder

Water to blend (optional)

288 calories
11 g fat
16 g carbs
4 g fiber
8 g sugar
31 g protein

CHERRY BOMB

If you can find them, use tart cherries. They're grown exclusively in Michigan, but a 12-week study found that animals fed tart cherries showed a 9 percent belly fat reduction over those fed a standard diet.

¾ cup frozen cherries

½ frozen banana

1 cup unsweetened almond milk

⅓ cup vanilla plant-based protein powder

½ cup ice cubes

Water to blend (optional)

The rule of apple nutrition: Synthetic fertilizers promote water retention, so the bigger the apple, the more diluted its nutrients. Smaller fruits give you more nutritional bang for your buck.

300 calories
3 g fat
38 g carbs
5 g fiber
19 g sugar
29 g protein

CHOCOLATE-COVERED APPLE

1 medium apple

1 tablespoon almonds

1 date

½ cup unsweetened almond milk

⅓ cup chocolate plant-based protein powder

½ cup ice cubes

Water to blend (optional)

294 calories
5 g fat
36 g carbs
7 g fiber
24 g sugar
28 g protein

SPICE THINGS UP

"Pepper greens" are a hot new grocery trend. Usually a mix of arugula, mustard greens, nasturtium, and other spicy lettuces, they add a surprise kick and a big dose of folate. Ginger adds its own spicy flavor, along with its antioxidant and anti-inflammatory powers.

1 cup pepper greens

1 teaspoon chopped fresh ginger

1 medium apple

2 teaspoons ground flaxseed

½ cup unsweetened almond milk

⅓ cup plant-based chocolate protein powder

½ cup ice cubes

Water to blend (optional)

Perfect garnish: a nasturtium flower

271 calories
6 g fat
31 g carbs
9 g fiber
19 g sugar
27 g protein

"HOT" CHOCOLATE

The heat from the cayenne makes the chocolate flavor pop.

1 tablespoon cacao powder

¼ avocado

1 cup ice

1 teaspoon cayenne pepper

1 cup unsweetened almond milk

1 scoop chocolate plant-based protein powder

295 calories
15 g fat
16 g carbs
8 g fiber
3 g sugar
29 g protein

APPLE AND PEANUT BUTTER

The after-school classic gets a twist that adults and kids will love.

1 teaspoon peanut butter

½ Pink Lady apple

½ frozen banana

1 cup unsweetened almond milk

1 scoop chocolate plant-based protein powder

3 ice cubes

Water to blend

303 calories
9 g fat
38 g carbs
11 g fiber
17 g sugar
20 g protein

CHAI OF THE TIGER

Chai is black tea that arrives in your belly with a posse. That posse is a collection of herbs and spices, all of which have their own superpowers, and can help you fight the battle for your health on numerous fronts. Chai improves immunity; fights inflammation; slows aging; and enhances cardiovascular functioning. Bonus: one sip whisks you away to aromatic India.

1 cup vanilla chai tea, cooled

1 cup spinach

½ frozen banana

1 teaspoon chia seeds

½ cup unsweetened almond milk

1 scoop chocolate plant-based protein powder

3 ice cubes

Water to blend

223 calories
2.6 g fat
22 g carbs
5 g fiber
10 g sugar
27.5 g protein

AB OF STEEL

One of my favorite almond butters is Justin's. It's made with dry-roasted almonds and a bit of sustainably-sourced palm fruit oil, which lends the spread its creamy texture. (They also make all-natural peanut butter cups that will make you question everything you thought you knew about the PB-chocolate combo.)

¾ frozen banana

2 teaspoons almond butter

¾ cup unsweetened almond milk

1 scoop chocolate or vanilla plant-based protein powder

340 calories
15 g fat
36 g carbs
10 g fiber
13 g sugar
20 g protein

ZERO BELLY TIP:

GO BANANAS FOR BANANAS.

One recent study found that women who ate a banana twice daily as a pre-meal snack for 60 days reduced their belly-bloat by 50 percent! Why? The fruit increases bloat-fighting bacteria in the stomach. Bananas are a terrific source of of potassium, which can help diminish retention of fluids.

8

SAVORY
SMOOTHIES

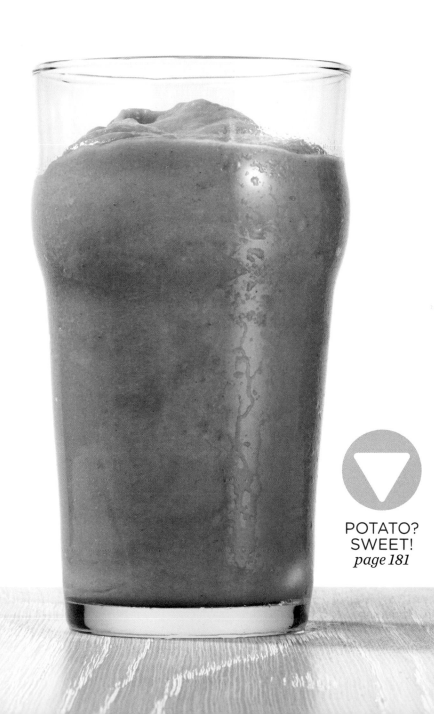

POTATO?
SWEET!
page 181

A smoothie can be a lot of things: a pre- or post-workout boost, a cold and refreshing thirst quencher, a thick and creamy dessert, a perfectly balanced breakfast. But one thing most of us never think of when we think of smoothies: comfort food.

These recipes stake out a new territory in the smoothie landscape, a culinary point of departure into a taste realm you might not have considered. While these smoothies are still cold and refreshing, they're going to taste more like a savory soup than a bright pick-me-up. And that's fine. If you follow the Zero Belly 7-Day Smoothie Cleanse at the end of this book, these are the perfect go-to flavors for lunchtime indulgence.

TURMERICAN DREAM

Turmeric may be the single most powerful anti-inflammatory food in nature's arsenal, thanks to its unique active compound, curcumin.
It's a staple of Indian food, and blends perfectly with tropical fruits like pineapple.

1 cup fresh pineapple, chunked

½ frozen banana

1 teaspoon turmeric

½ cup unsweetened almond milk

1 scoop plant-based plain protein powder

293 calories
3 g fat
43 g carbs
6 g fiber
26 g sugar
27 g protein

CARROT TOP

This one's a fresh smoothie perfect for fall, with an eye-opening kick of ginger that lasts year-round.

2 carrots, peeled

½ frozen banana

1 cup unsweetened almond milk

1 teaspoon fresh ginger, grated

1 scoop vanilla plant-based protein powder

1 teaspoon ground flaxseed

295 calories
5 g fat
36 g carbs
7 g fiber
16 g sugar
28 g protein

TEST PANEL FAVORITE!

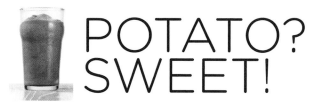

POTATO? SWEET!

Bananas and sweet potatoes both add starch, but that's why the cinnamon is in there. Adding cinnamon to a starchy meal helps stabilize blood sugar and ward off insulin spikes, according to a series of studies printed in *The American Journal of Clinical Nutrition*.

½ **cooked sweet potato,** cooled, with skin off

½ **frozen banana**

½ **teaspoon cinnamon**

1 cup unsweetened almond milk

1 scoop plain plant-based protein powder

280 calories
5 g fat
34 g carbs
6 g fiber
14 g sugar
28 g protein

BIG RED

Beets provide a solid dose of the nutrient betaine, which turns off the genes for insulin resistance and abdominal fat gain. Buy them whole and save (and cook) the greens; they score higher than even spinach on the nutritional density score.

1 cooked beet

1 tablespoon almond butter

1 teaspoon coconut oil

½ cup unsweetened almond milk

1 scoop plant-based plain protein powder

3 ice cubes

Water to blend (recommended for this one)

305 calories
10 g fat
41 g carbs
8 g fiber
4 g sugar
26 g protein

BASIL QUINOA

All the protein of power of quinoa, none of the chewing.

½ cup cooked quinoa, cooled

3 basil leaves

1 cup unsweetened almond milk

1 scoop plant-based plain protein powder

honey to taste

331 calories
6 g fat
35 g carbs
5 g fiber
3 g sugar
32 g protein

TABASCO CHERRY

This one has a kick to it, softened by the cherry aftertaste.

½ **cup cherries**

½ **frozen banana**

1 tsp Tabasco sauce

¼ **lime**

¼ **cup unsweetened almond milk**

1 scoop plant-based plain protein powder

3 ice cubes

Water to blend (optional)

232 calories
2 g fat
28 g carbs
3.5 g fiber
10 g sugar
26 g protein

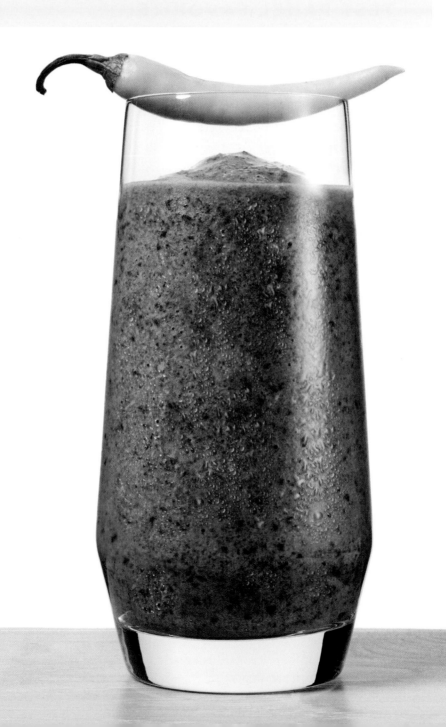

MR. BEAN

You won't even taste the secret ingredient here.

¼ **cup kidney beans**

½ **frozen banana**

½ **cup frozen strawberries**

4 mint leaves

1 cup unsweetened almond milk

¼ **scoop plant-based plain protein powder**

340 calories
4.5 g fat
53 g carbs
11 g fiber
14 g sugar
24 g protein

GARLIC APPLE

Your doctor is going to have to go find some new patients. A powerful anti-inflammatory agent, garlic also seems to reduce the risk of gastro-intestinal disease, according to the National Cancer Institute. Don't worry: you don't put it in the Smoothie.

¼ apple

¼ avocado

¼ cup cucumber

1 cup unsweetened almond milk

1 scoop plant-based plain protein powder

dash of garlic powder

3 ice cubes

304 calories
14 g fat
19 g carbs
7 g fiber
8 g sugar
27 g protein

PUMPKIN SPICE

Unlike the pumpkin spice lattes you love, this drink has actual pumpkin in it. One-third cup of pumpkin provides protein, fiber, omega-3 fatty acids, and 16% of your recommended daily intake of vitamin C—a nutrient researchers say is directly related to the body's ability to burn through fat. In fact, one study by researchers from Arizona State University showed deficiencies of vitamin C were strongly correlated with increased body fat and waist measurements.

½ **frozen banana**

⅓ **cup pumpkin puree**

¼ **teaspoon pumpkin spice**

⅛ **teaspoon vanilla extract**

1 **teaspoon flax seeds**

1 **cup unsweetened almond milk**

1 **scoop plant-based plain protein powder**

292 calories
5 g fat
33 g carbs
7 g fiber
14 g sugar
29 g protein

CHICK-FIL-O

The sneaky source of extra protein here: the chickpeas.

¼ cup cooked rolled oats

⅛ cup chickpeas

sprig of cilantro

1 cup unsweetened almond milk

1 scoop plain plant-based protein powder

277 calories
6 g fat
26 g carbs
6 g fiber
4 g sugar
20 g protein

RED PEPPER PUNCH

You can't go wrong here:
Add even more pepper if it's
not red enough.

¼ **red bell pepper**

½ **tomato**

1 celery stick

1 dash cayenne pepper

½ **cup unsweetened almond milk**

1 scoop plant-based plain protein powder

170 calories
2 g fat
10 g carbs
3 g fiber
5 g sugar
26 g protein

TEST PANEL FAVORITE!

FALL HARVEST

The nutty, roasted flavor of green tea steps in brilliantly here as a base for a delicious smoothie that will have you reminiscing about the Thanksgivings of your childhood.

½ **cooked sweet potato,** cooled, with skin off

½ **banana**

⅛ **teaspoon nutmeg**

½ **teaspoon cinnamon**

6 medium-sized basil leaves

¼ **cup green tea**

1 cup unsweetened almond milk

1 scoop plain plant-based protein powder

283 calories
5 g fat
35 g carbs
7 g fiber
14 g sugar
28 g protein

STUFFED SWEET POTATO

Is this a Thanksgiving side dish or a smoothie? Either way, it makes for a delicious lunchtime treat.

¼ **cooked sweet potato,** cold

¼ **teaspoon thyme**

1 tablespoon chia seeds

1 cup unsweetened almond milk

1 scoop plant-based plain protein powder

230 calories
7 g fat
17 g carbs
6 g fiber
4.6 g sugar
28 g protein

SWAP SUGARY DRINKS FOR A SMOOTHIE!

Be sure your drinks don't have added sugar. Elevated glucose and fructose in your body weakens collagen and elastin, the structural supports that keep skin tight and plump. The sugar links to amino acids in the skin to produce advanced glycation end products, whose acronym "AGEs" aptly describes what they do to skin. The process is accelerated by ultraviolet light, according to a study in *Clinical Dermatology*. In other words, eating lots of sugar poolside is the worst thing you can do for your skin.

CHAPTER

9

NUTRITIONIST FAVORITES!

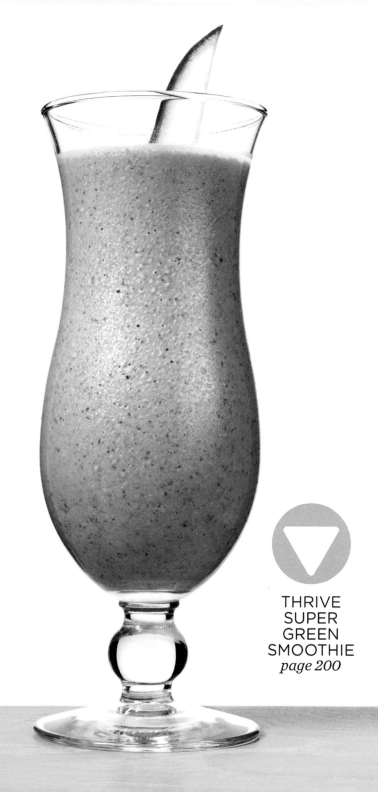

THRIVE
SUPER
GREEN
SMOOTHIE
page 200

The wonderful thing about the Zero Belly Superfoods is, there's so much variety, it's just fun to mix and match them. For this chapter, I asked the country's top nutritionists to share with me their favorite plant-based smoothie, keeping the foods in mind, and the results are all delicious and nutritious. Pay attention to the protein counts—if it's under 25 grams, you don't want them as a meal replacement, but rather paired with a meal.

All recipes serve one unless otherwise indicated.

CHOCOLATE PEANUT BUTTER

by Gina Hassick, MA, RD, LDN, CDE, NCC and owner of Eat Well with Gina (eatwellwithgina.com)

1 handful spinach

1 handful baby kale

1 cup chocolate soy milk

1 small frozen banana

1 tablespoon All-Natural Peanut Butter

Ice

"This Chocolate Peanut Butter Smoothie is my go-to non-dairy smoothie because it is decadent, yet nutritious—the best of both worlds. The combination of chocolate and peanut butter creates a rich flavor to satisfy your sweet tooth, but the spinach, kale and protein from the soy milk help to create a balance to keep blood sugars steady. This smoothie is also a nutritional powerhouse packed with immune boosting nutrients like vitamin C and potassium and is packed with fiber to help keep you feeling fuller for longer and help aid in weight loss goals."

Per 1 serving:
346 calories
13 g fat
47 g carbs
7 g fiber
23 g sugar
15 g protein

WAKE-UP CALL

by Kristin Reisinger, MS, RD, CSSD and founder and owner of IronPlate Studios

½ cup frozen mixed berries

Handful of spinach

8 oz unsweetened Silk almond milk

1 scoop plant-based vanilla protein powder
(Reisinger uses VegaOne Vanilla Performance Protein)

"Combining a low-calorie, non-dairy smoothie first thing in the morning with a roughly even portion of high-quality protein and good carbs is a great start to anyone looking to lose weight and be healthy. Starting the day off with a smoothie such as this will pull your body out of it's overnight fasting state, and the carbohydrates from healthy, mixed berries combined with high-quality protein will give you the quick energy and protein uptake your body needs first thing in the morning without being 'too much.'"

Per 1 serving:
230 calories
2.5 g fat
20 g carbs
5 g fiber
7 g sugar
26 g protein

PEANUT BUTTER AND JELLY

by Jim White, RD, ACSM HFS, and owner of
Jim White Fitness and Nutrition Studios

¾ cup berries
(blueberries, blackberries, raspberries)

1 tablespoon nut butter, natural

1 cup unsweetened almond milk

1 scoop plain plant-based protein powder

Per 1 serving:
328 calories
12 g fat
24 g carbs
7 g fiber
11 g sugar
30 g protein

"Who doesn't love a PB and J sandwich! Well, now you can have the same experience without the extra bread. This non-dairy smoothie is not only delicious but quite nutritious. It can be a great on-the-go breakfast option, consumed as a snack or post-work-out. It provides a powerful punch of protein, fiber, antioxidants, essential fats and vital nutrients to support good health."

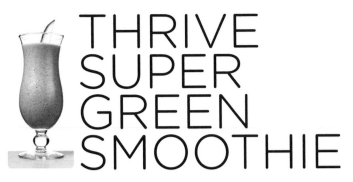

THRIVE SUPER GREEN SMOOTHIE

by Katie Cavuto, MS, RD

½ cup raw coconut water

1 cups greens (spinach, kale, arugula, etc**)**

¼ cucumber

¼ apple, cored

¼ banana

¼ lemon, juiced (zest optional)

½ teaspoon orange zest

1 tablespoons hemp seeds

½ tablespoon ground flax

**½ tablespoon nut butter or
   2 tablespoons nuts**

Water to thin to desired consistency

200 calories
15 g fat
25 g carbs
5 g fiber
16 g sugar
7 g protein

"While it may seem easy and taste great to load your blender with heaps of fruit, I often remind my clients to balance their smoothie like they would any other meal. A well-balanced smoothies contains a blend of fruit with other nutrient dense ingredients like healthy fats, proteins and vegetables. This smoothie has it all—the least of which is fruit! Greens pair with satisfying fats and proteins from nuts and seeds which are sweetened naturally by the fruit and citrus zest. It is refreshing and satiating."

Adapted from "The Nourished Green Smoothie" on Nourish.Breathe.Thrive.

APPLE SPICE SMOOTHIE

by Miriam Jacobson, RD, CDN

1 apple

Handful of kale, deveined

1 teaspoon matcha powder

1 cup unsweetened almond milk

1 scoop plain plant-based protein powder

cinnamon and nutmeg to taste

"This apple spice smoothie is a favorite breakfast of mine. I almost always have all the ingredients at home, which makes it a no-hassle recipe—not to mention that the combination is beyond delicious. The cinnamon balances blood sugar levels, curbing the appetite and preventing aimless snacking throughout the morning hours. Plus the matcha powder contains catechins like EGCG that help to stimulate fat loss from storage sites. Drink up!"

300 calories
4.5 g fat
40 g carbs
8 g fiber
21 g sugar
28 g protein

THE CARB-CUTTER

by Amy Shapiro MS, RD, CDN

¾ cup frozen berries

½ cup frozen spinach

1 tablespoon chia seeds

Dash of cinnamon

Dash of turmeric

1 cup unsweetened almond milk

1 scoop vanilla plant-based protein powder

"I love this protein shake because it's loaded with nutrients but void of excess calories and sugar. I recommend berries as they are high in fiber, low in calories and loaded with disease fighting antioxidants—and chia seeds add 'staying power' as they help to keep you full and provide tons of omega 3 fatty acids. The cinnamon helps to balance blood sugar levels and may help with weight loss and almond milk has fewer calories than cow's milk and a mild flavor that adds 5 grams of heart-healthy fat but not extra carbs!"

267 calories
7 g fat
24 g carbs
9 g fiber
10 g sugar
29 g protein

RASPBERRY CHOCOLATE SMOOTHIE

by Isabel Smith, MS, RD, CDN

½ banana

1 handful spinach

½ cup raspberries

1 tablespoon almond or cashew nut butter

2 tablespoons raw cocoa powder

10 oz unsweetened almond, hemp or coconut milk

1 scoop or serving plant-based protein powder (optional)

Without scoop of protein:

257 calories
15 g fat
32 g carbs
11 g fiber
10 g sugar
8.6 g protein

With scoop of protein:

391 calories
15 g fat
38 g carbs
12 g fiber
12 g sugar
34 g protein

"I really love this smoothie because it tastes super-decadent, but in reality is just loaded with a ton of natural, unprocessed and healthful ingredients."

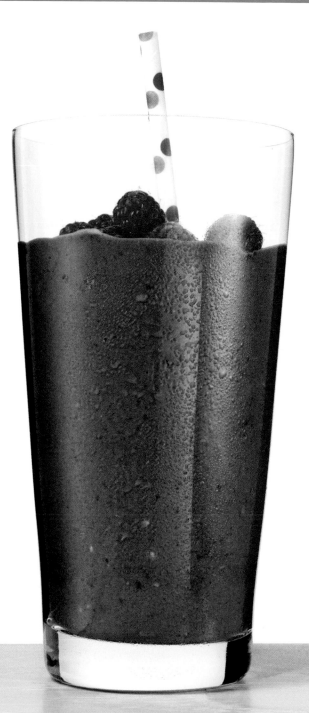

APPLE-CABBAGE SMOOTHIE

by Sarah Koszyk, MA, RDN, Registered Dietitian/Nutritionist & Founder of Family. Food. Fiesta.

1 small green apple (cored and cubed)

¾ cup purple cabbage (roughly chopped)

½ cup frozen blueberries

1 tablespoon chia seeds

½ cup coconut water or regular water

"I love this smoothie because it's packed with vitamin C and omega-3s, making it a superfood winner for overall health. Both blueberries and purple cabbage contain vitamin C, which are great for glowing skin. The chia seeds have omega-3s perfect for brain and heart health. When I'm low in energy and need a boost, I go to this smoothie for a complete pick-me-up. It helps keep me nourished, fueled, and satiated with a balance of protein, fruit, vegetables, and fat to control hunger levels and keep me strong."

245 calories
5 g fat
45 g carbs
13 g fiber
27 g sugar
7 g protein

GREEN VEGGIE SMOOTHIE

by Isabel Smith, MS, RD, CDN

Pair this with some eggs for an A.M. treat.

1 small pear, cored

1 kiwi, peeled

1 cucumber, chopped

¼ avocado

1-inch ginger, peeled

½ lemon, juiced

1 handful spinach

4 oz water (can be replaced for unsweetened, plain coconut water)

307 calories
11 g fat
54 g carbs
13 g fiber
26 g sugar
6 g protein

"I love this smoothie because it's refreshing, yet packed with nutrients like vitamin C, heart-healthy potassium, and antioxidants like quercetin, beta-carotene, and gingerol. And because it's got anti-inflammatory and heart-healthy avocado, I love to have it for breakfast because the fat helps to slow digestion, keeping me fuller for longer."

KALE RECHARGE SMOOTHIE

by Lyssie Lakatos, RDN, CDN, CFT and
Tammy Lakatos Shames, RD, CDN, CFT

With such a low protein count,
this smoothie wouldn't qualify as a meal
replacement, but it does pair well
with an omelet, as the nutritionists
suggest. Serves 3.

1 frozen, very ripe banana

¾ cup spinach, loosely packed

¾ cups curly kale, stems removed, loosely packed

½ cup carrots, chopped

1 teaspoon ginger, grated

1 tablespoon fresh parsley (or cilantro)

1 teaspoon lime juice

8 ounces water

4 ice cubes

"This easy-to-make smoothie is our go-to when we want an extra lift; it's a simple way to get restorative, nutrient rich green veggies in the morning that flood the body with phytonutrients to prevent destructive toxins and inflammation from harming the body. The fiber helps to flush waste from the colon for a flatter stomach, while the fluid and potassium help to hydrate your skin and body, restoring normal fluid balance and flushing bloating sodium, 'de-puffing' you and making you feel lighter. At just 58 calories, this smoothie helps to fill you up and take the edge off hunger helping to keep you lean and svelte. Pair it with a veggie omelet for a satisfying, healthy breakfast."

Per serving:
58 calories
0 g fat
14 g carbs
3 g fiber
5 g sugar
2 g protein

BANANA FUDGE SMOOTHIE

by Cheryl Forberg, RD, and author of
A Small Guide to Losing Big

¾ cups very cold vanilla soymilk

¼ cup soft silken tofu

1 ripe medium banana,
    frozen and cut into 1-inch chunks

1 tablespoon unsweetened natural cocoa powder

½ teaspoon agave nectar

"Creamy and delicious, this smoothie is great for breakfast or a midday pick-me-up."

247 calories
4.6 g fat
46 g carbs
6 g fiber
27 g sugar
9 g protein

With permission from **A Small Guide to Losing Big** by Cheryl Forberg RD (Flavor First Publishing 2015)

CASSETTA'S PUMPKIN PIE

by Jennifer Cassetta, clinical nutritionist, personal trainer

1 cup canned pumpkin

1 cup coconut or almond milk

1 teaspoon pumpkin pie spice

½ banana

2 tablespoons of chopped pecans

¾ scoop Vega Vanilla protein powder

Handful of ice cubes

331 calories
10 g fat
42 g carbs
11 g fiber
17 g sugar
24 g protein

"Pumpkin pie without the pie, all year round? Yes please! Pumpkin is a good clean burning carbohydrate and when you add the protein powder you'll balance your blood sugar as well as add the perfect components for a post workout recovery meal."

TROPICAL SMOOTHIE

by Leah Kaufman, MS, RD, CDN

½ cup spinach

½ banana

1 cup frozen fruit:
mangoes, pineapple, strawberries

1 cup coconut water

Pair this with a high-protein meal for a vitamin-packed breakfast and lunch. "This smoothie is perfect for when you are missing the summer weather. The tropical smoothie provides you with iron, vitamin C, potassium, and more. Not only does it have amazing benefits, it also tastes great!"

148 calories
1 g fat
34 g carbs
7 g fiber
20 g sugar
4 g protein

CINNAMON BANANA

by Lisa Moskovitz, RD, CDN

½ **banana**

1 tablespoon of ground chia seeds

1 teaspoon of cinnamon powder

1 cup of light vanilla almond milk

1 scoop of plant-based protein powder

262 calories
4 g fat
32 g carbs
4.4 g fiber
20 g sugar
27 g protein

"Sometimes life doesn't give you the opportunity to sit down and have a solid meal, so having a satisfying, yet nutritious, go-to smoothie recipe is a must. This creamy and refreshing dairy-free smoothie has two of the best nutrients for slashing hunger and keeping calories low: 14g of lean protein + 7g of fiber."

CREAMY CHOCOLATE PEANUT BUTTER

by Stephanie Clark R.D., Willow Jarosh, R.D of C&J Nutrition

8-10 ounces unsweetened almond milk

¾ medium, very ripe banana

1 tablespoon peanut butter

¼ cup cubed soft tofu

1 heaping cups steamed and cooled cauliflower florets

½ tablespoon cocoa powder
  (Use more if you want it super chocolate-y)

¹⁄₁₆ teaspoon cinnamon

Small handful ice cubes

300 calories
19 g fat
36 g carbs
12 g fiber
16 g sugar
15 g protein

Place all ingredients, except for ice into a blender and blend on high for 1 to 1½ minutes, until mixture is smooth. Then add ice and blend for an addition 1 to 1½ minutes until mixture is smooth.

Although tofu isn't a Zero Belly Diet food, because it may lead to bloating, I love how Stephanie and Willow got creative by adding it to increase the protein count here. If you show no sensitivities to tofu, enjoy this one guilt-free.

BEET-CHERRY

by Dana James MS, CNS, CDN, BANT, AADP,
Founder of Food Coach NYC & LA

10 oz unsweetened almond milk

1 raw beet

1 cup frozen cherries

1 teaspoon hemp seeds

3 tablespoons Beauti-Fuel brand protein powder

Dash of Belgarian Rose Water

"I borrowed this recipe from my dear friend, Rebecca Leffler's, book Très Green, Très Clean, Très Chic. *She paired the unusual combination of beets and cherries and it worked beautifully —earthiness juxtaposed against sweetness. I added some hemp seeds and a dash of rose water help intensify the skin's radiance."*

239 calories
6.5 g fat
35 g carbs
8.6 g fiber
23 g sugar
15 g protein

COCONUT CASHEW PROTEIN SMOOTHIE

by Cassie Bjork, RD, LD of Healthy Simple Life

½ banana

1 tablespoon of cashew butter

¼ cup full-fat coconut milk

2 scoops dairy-free PaleoMeal protein powder

1 scoop of Espresso Dynamic Greens

2-3 ice cubes

315 calories
21 g fat
26 g carbs
4 g fiber
9 g sugar
14 g protein

"This is my go-to smoothie recipe for weight loss because it contains a balance of protein, fat and carbs which promote stable blood sugar levels and in turn, your pancreas can secrete your fat-burning hormone, glucagon! And it's so good, you can drink one every morning and not get sick of it!"

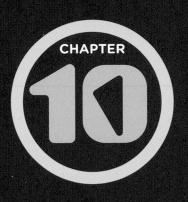

CHAPTER

10

THE ZERO BELLY 7-DAY SMOOTHIE CLEANSE

Doing nothing more than swapping a few Zero Belly Smoothies into your day will result in dramatic weight loss. But you can take your results to the next level by following the Zero Belly 7-Day Cleanse and increasing your smoothie intake to create an effective plan that will flatten your belly in record time.

If you're already following the Zero Belly program, then you've no doubt seen for yourself how powerful it can be. But if you're new to it, here's a quick look at the overall program.

HOW THE ZERO BELLY DIET WORKS

The science of Zero Belly is the science of flavor.

This is a weight-loss plan that focuses on taste, because the taste of a food is the single strongest indicator that it has the power to unlock your metabolism, heal your body, even turn off the genes responsible for weight gain. Sweet, moist fruits; deep, decadent chocolate; bright, crunchy vegetables; and rich, silky oils are the backbone of the Zero Belly plan, each enhanced with herbs and spices that are as potent on your plate and in your glass as they are inside your body. Zero Belly Smoothies harness the power of real food to target belly fat—the most dangerous type of fat there is—by unlocking your body's own natural fat burners.

Here's a quick rundown of the Zero Belly foods and how each of them will inform the drink recipes in this book.

ZERO BELLY SMOOTHIES
Maximize Nutritional Intake

The original Zero Belly program included one blended smoothie drink per day. If you're currently enjoying success with Zero Belly, then this book has no doubt provided a whole new set of recipes to inform your palate and delight your taste buds. But if you want to turbocharge your results, the cleanse outlined in this chapter will show you how to strip away belly fat even faster. Studies show that high-protein, low-fat smoothies are highly effective at rushing nutrients into your body, particularly your muscles.

A reminder: I've stripped all the Zero Belly Smoothie recipes of dairy, added sugars, and artificial ingredients so common in popular commercial shakes, and packed them with real fruits, nuts, vegan proteins, and dairy alternatives like almond and coconut milks. Why the alternative milks? First, dairy can be difficult to digest for some folks—and poor digestion leads to inflammation, which leads to weight gain. But there's more to it than that: In 2014, Swedish scientists at Uppsala University found that women who drank three or more glasses of milk a day died at nearly twice the rate of those who drank less than one glass a day. Broken bones were more common in women who were heavy milk drinkers as well. While this is only a preliminary study, it's further reason why using nondairy milk in your daily smoothie is a wise move.

Eggs
Turn Off Visceral Fat Genes

Eggs are the single best dietary source of the B vitamin choline, an essential nutrient used in the construction of all the body's cell membranes. Choline deficiency is linked directly to the genes that cause visceral fat accumulation, particularly in the liver. Yet according to a 2015 National Health and Nutrition Examination Survey, only a small percentage of all Americans eat daily diets that meet the U.S. Institute of Medicine's Adequate Intake of 425 milligrams for women and 550 milligrams for men.

Of course, unless you're filming yet another sequel to

Rocky, drinking raw eggs isn't in your nutrition plan. But while there are no egg-smoothie recipes, you should make an effort to include them in your diet as often as you can.

RED FRUIT
Turn Off Obesity Genes

Like professional basketball players, all fruits are good at what they do. But a red hue is a sign that your snack is just that little bit better—watermelon is to honeydew what LeBron James is to a backup on the Knicks. And since the release of *Zero Belly Diet,* more and more evidence keeps proving that point. For example, a study in the journal *Evolution and Human Behaviour* found that people who ate more portions of red and orange fruits and vegetables had a more sun-kissed complexion than those who ate less—the result of disease-fighting compounds called carotenoids. You'll find a wide array of red fruits used throughout the drink recipes in this book.

ZERO BELLY FAVORITES:
ruby red grapefruit, tart cherries, raspberries, strawberries, blueberries, blackberries, red apples (especially Pink Lady), watermelon, plums, peaches, nectarines

OLIVE OIL AND OTHER HEALTHY FATS
Vanquish Hunger

Fat does more than just make our food taste good. In fact, the right kinds of fat, like that found in olive oil, nuts, and avocados, can ward off the munchies by regulating hunger hormones. A study published in *Nutrition Journal* found that participants who ate half a fresh avocado with lunch reported a 40 percent decreased desire to eat for hours afterward. And a brand-new study by scientists in India looked at 60 middle-aged men who were at risk for diabetes and heart disease. They gave the two groups similar diets, except that one of these groups got 20 percent of their daily calories from pistachios. The group of men who ate the pistachios had smaller waists at the end of the study period; their cholesterol score dropped by an average of 15 points, and their blood sugar numbers improved as well.

You may not think of fats as an ingredient in a drink, but dietary fat is essential to creating a drink that will strip away body fat. You'll find healthy fats from sources like avocados, nut butters, and coconut throughout the recipes in this book.

ZERO BELLY FAVORITES:

extra-virgin olive oil, virgin coconut oil, avocados, walnuts, cashews, almonds, almond butter, wild salmon, sardines, ground flaxseed (flax meal), chia seeds

BEANS, RICE, OATS, AND OTHER HEALTHY FIBER
Turn Off Diabetes Genes

Think of beans as little weight-loss pills and enjoy them whenever you'd like. One study found that people who ate ¾ cup of beans daily weighed 6.6 pounds less than those who didn't, even though the bean eaters consumed, on average, 199 more calories per day. Part of the reason is that fiber—from beans and whole grains—helps our bodies (okay, actually the bacteria in our bodies) produce a substance called butyrate, which deactivates the genes that cause insulin insensitivity.

One common source of fiber that you won't find in these recipes, however, is wheat. Zero Belly isn't specifically a gluten-free program, but all the recipes in this book are gluten-free for a reason: If you have gluten intolerance, then this protein will cause inflammation in your gut. My goal has been to create a plan that will work for *everyone*. So go ahead and have your Wheaties if you want, but more and more science says that sticking with the Zero Belly fiber sources might make more sense: According to a study in the *Annals of Nutrition and Metabolism,* scientists found that having oatmeal (in this case, Quaker Oats Quick 1-Minute Oats) for breakfast resulted in greater fullness, lower hunger ratings, and fewer calories eaten at the next meal compared with a serving of ready-to-eat sugared cornflakes, even though the calorie counts of the two breakfasts were identical.

In fact, fiber causes you to lose weight even if you do absolutely nothing else to improve your diet. In a study at the University of South Carolina, subjects who ate an average of 16.6 grams of fiber per day were put on diets that increased their fiber intake to an average of 28.4 grams a day, while eating the same number of calories and not exercising at all. After four weeks, the subjects had lost an average of 3 pounds each, and both groups reported less hunger and more satiety. This despite the fact that the subjects didn't exercise or take any other steps toward weight loss other than to boost their fiber.

ZERO BELLY FAVORITES:
peanuts and peanut butter, old-fashioned oats, quinoa, brown rice, canned black and garbanzo beans, French green lentils, peas

EXTRA PROTEIN
Boosts Metabolism

One of the unique qualities of Zero Belly is its reliance on plant-based proteins. While I'm no vegetarian—not by a long shot!—I also know that relying on dairy-based supplements to boost your protein intake isn't always the best bet for those of us focused on balancing our gut health, especially those who suffer from lactose intolerance.

And more and more research is showing that when we add plant proteins to our diets, our bodies respond by shedding fat. In a 2015 study in the *Journal of Diabetes Investigation,* researchers discovered that patients who ingested higher amounts of vegetable protein were far less susceptible to metabolic syndrome (a disease that ought to be renamed "diabolic syndrome"—it's basically a combination of high cholesterol, high blood sugar, and obesity). That means eating whole foods from vegetables—and supplementing with vegan protein powder—is one of the best ways to keep extra weight at bay. A second study in *Nutrition Journal* found that "plant protein intakes may play a role in preventing obesity."

Zero Belly Smoothies are made specifically with plant protein, but to add more into your day, focus on vegetable protein sources like lentils, hemp or chia seeds, quinoa, nuts, seeds, and beans. Or try adding spirulina to your smoothies; it's one of the few plant foods that are mostly protein by weight (about 70 percent).

ZERO BELLY FAVORITES:
Vega One All-in-One Nutritional Shake; Vega Sport Performance Protein; Sunwarrior Warrior Blend

LEAN MEATS AND FISH

Build Muscle and Turn Off Fat-Storage Genes

Maintaining and building muscle is important, especially as we get older. Increased muscle mass means a healthier weight, better fitness, and improved quality of life. But in order to get those benefits, we may need to eat more protein than we currently do. A lot of this can come from plant proteins in our Zero Belly Smoothies. But an extra helping of lean meat might not be a bad idea, either. In a 2015 study in the *American Journal of Physiology—Endocrinology and Metabolism*, researchers found that those who ate twice as much protein as the RDA had greater net protein balance and muscle protein synthesis—in other words, it was easier for them to maintain and build muscle. (Interestingly, the researchers found that it didn't matter when you ate the protein, just that you ate it.)

ZERO BELLY FAVORITES:

boneless skinless chicken breast, lean ground turkey (94 percent), lean beef, lamb, wild salmon, shrimp, scallops, cod, tuna, halibut, orange roughy, freshwater fish (like pike and sunfish)

LEAFY GREENS, GREEN TEA, AND BRIGHT VEGETABLES

Stop Inflammation and Turn Off Fat-Storage Genes

A leafy green like Swiss chard is a veritable Swiss Army knife for weight loss, which is why vegetables, as well as fruits, show up in many of the delicious recipes in this book. When you eat more greens, you arm your body with high levels of folate, a B vitamin that's been linked to everything from boosting mood to battling cancer. It's also a key that locks down genes linked to insulin resistance and fat-cell formation.

But leafy greens also perform another important function: They help provide you with a healthy, balanced gut. See, it's not enough to just get beneficial bacteria into your body. To make sure the good guys stay healthy and thrive, you need to feed them. And what they really love is something called fructooligosaccharides, or FOS, a type of fiber found in vegetables as well as fruits and grains. But veggies, because of their low caloric load, are probably the healthiest way of all to get these essential nutrients into your belly. FOS has been shown to increase absorption of vitamins and minerals, improve feelings of fullness, and otherwise keep everything running "clean."

ZERO BELLY FAVORITES:
watercress, Chinese cabbage, spinach, romaine, kale, carrots, Swiss chard, zucchini, red bell peppers, grape tomatoes, mesclun greens, leafy green herbs (parsley, oregano, basil, rosemary)

YOUR FAVORITE SPICES
Turn Off Genes for Inflammation and Weight Gain

Herbs, spices, and flavorings do more than add extra pizzazz to your food. From battling cancer to managing insulin response to fighting inflammation, many of the spices that sit on your pantry shelf are secret nutritional superstars, and the more you can incorporate them into your daily meals and Zero Belly Smoothies, the better. Spices and herbs are among the most powerful anti-inflammatory agents in the food world, and when you dampen inflammation, you set the table for faster weight loss.

To test the actual potency of spices after they've been ingested, researchers at the University of Florida, Gainesville, and at Penn State had subjects eat significant amounts of different spices every day for a week. Then they tested the subjects' blood plasma by dripping it onto inflamed white blood cells. The plasma of subjects who ate cloves, ginger, rosemary, and turmeric were the most potent—in other words, these spices have the highest level of anti-inflammatory impact after ingestion.

That's exciting news. All four flavor enhancers are essential parts of the Zero Belly Smoothie recipes, but turmeric deserves special attention. It's one of the magical nutrients that have been shown to work directly on our fat genes, turning off the specific genetic mechanism that's responsible for inflammation and obesity. In a 2015 study in the journal *Clinical Nutrition*, researchers gave 117 patients with metabolic syndrome either supplements of curcumin—the active ingredient in turmeric—or a placebo. Over eight weeks, those who received the curcumin saw dramatic reductions in inflammation and fasting blood sugar. Another reason why this spice belongs in your pantry.

ZERO BELLY FAVORITES:

yellow mustard, black pepper, turmeric, cinnamon, raw apple cider vinegar, dark chocolate with a cacao content of 70 percent or higher

HOW TO FOLLOW THE ZERO BELLY 7-DAY SMOOTHIE CLEANSE

The Zero Belly 7-Day Smoothie Cleanse is nothing more than a simple tweaking of the standard Zero Belly Diet. It's just a little more intense, because you're replacing two meals a day with drinks.

The plan is simple: You'll enjoy two Zero Belly Smoothies as meals (breakfast and lunch), two snacks, and a Zero Belly dinner. On the regular plan, you'd have three meals and two snacks, with one of those snacks being a drink. Here, I'm replacing both breakfast and lunch with drinks, which will cut your daily calories just a bit. (Note: If you'd prefer to eat breakfast and drink dinner, be my guest. I suggest breakfast and lunch because they tend to be the most harried times of the day, and hence a smoothie can help, er, smooth things out.)

How come? Since the drinks average about 300 calories each, this step alone will cut approximately 500 to 1,000 calories out of your daily intake, which may take several additional pounds off your body in just seven days. The drinks pack such a nutritional punch that I know you'll be getting the vitamins, minerals, protein, and healthy fats you need. Remember to always ask the three Zero Belly questions before each drink, meal, or snack:

WHERE'S MY PROTEIN?
WHERE'S MY FIBER?
WHERE'S MY HEALTHY FAT?

HOW TO BUILD A ZERO BELLY 7-DAY SMOOTHIE CLEANSE DINNER

If you're drinking breakfast and lunch, then having a full, satisfying dinner makes all the sense in the world. Here's how to create one that complements the Zero Belly Smoothies plan perfectly.

1
PICK YOUR PROTEIN

6 ounces chicken breast (skinless)

6 ounces lean ground turkey (at least 93 percent)

6 ounces lean ground beef (grass-fed, at least 90 percent)

6 ounces lean steak (grass-fed, sirloin, or anything labeled "round")

6 ounces fish (wild)

2-3 eggs

2
ADD A FIBER

Stop thinking in terms of carbs and instead think of fiber. Focus on gluten-free fiber sources to help fight inflammation and bloating.

Brown, black, or wild rice

Quinoa

Beans

Peas

Lentils

Spiced oatmeal

Grainful is a new line of "steel-cut meals," which can be served as side dishes or combined with meat into one dish. Flavors include Thai Curry, Cheddar Broccoli, and Vegetarian Chili. All weigh in at 6 grams of fiber or more. Pasta alternatives: Many companies have begun producing gluten-free pasta products out of high-fiber, high-protein foods. Check out Banza pasta, made from chickpeas (twice the protein and four times the fiber of regular pasta), or Tolerant, a line of bean- and lentil-based pastas, which are even more potent.

3

STEAM, STIR-FRY, OR BUILD A SIDE SALAD
With Some Combination of These Vegetables

(Note that cruciferous vegetables like kale, cabbage, broccoli, and cauliflower are not on the list, as they can cause bloating. Feel free to enjoy them if they don't irritate you, but I kept them off the recommended list just in case.)

Spinach

Romaine or other lettuce

Asparagus

Grape tomatoes

Carrots

Bell peppers

Mushrooms

Zucchini or squash

Herbs and spices

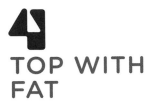

TOP WITH FAT

¼ avocado

2 tablespoons nuts/
seeds

Olive, walnut, avocado,
or hazelnut oil

Or top with this recipe for Zero Belly Vinaigrette.

ZERO BELLY VINAIGRETTE
Yield: 1 cup, about 16 servings

⅓ **cup apple cider vinegar**

⅔ **cup extra-virgin olive oil**

1½ **teaspoons Dijon mustard**

1½ **teaspoons honey**

¼ **teaspoon salt**

¼ **teaspoon fresh ground black pepper**

Combine ingredients in a mason jar
and shake vigorously until emulsified.
Store in fridge and shake before serving.

WHAT TO EXPECT IF YOU FOLLOW THE ZERO BELLY DIET

The 6-week Zero Belly Diet plan, as outlined in the *New York Times* bestseller, is just as simple to follow as the cleanse.

When I first assembled a test panel to prove the theories behind the Zero Belly program, I knew I was on to something exciting. I created a six-week test, figuring that subjects would almost certainly drop 5 to 10 percent of their body weight in that time.

But I wasn't prepared for how rapidly the panel saw results, and how dramatic those changes turned out to be. Here's a look at what happened:

WEEK

LOOK AND FEEL LIGHTER—IMMEDIATELY

The first thing you'll notice on this program—within a few days, in most cases—is that your pants will fit better, you'll look leaner, and you'll feel less bloated and lighter. You'll step on the scale and wonder if this is a trick; while you may lose up to 7 pounds in the first week, you'll feel like you've lost a lot more.

That's because the first thing Zero Belly affects is your digestion, helping balance your gut health, reduce bloating, and fight inflammation. It's step one in your attack on belly fat: You're prepping your body for dramatic weight loss. Your belly will almost immediately look leaner, and you'll notice a huge spike in energy and emotional well-being.

That's what Morgan Minor, a 24-year-old firefighter in Coalinga, California, told us. Within a week of starting the Zero Belly program she had dropped 7 pounds, and after just 21 days, a sculpted stomach emerged—Morgan had shed 4 inches off her waist by focusing on the Zero Belly foods and enjoying Zero Belly Smoothies. "My favorite was the Peanut Butter Sandwich," she says. (The recipe is in Chapter Seven.)

Bryan Wilson, 29, a bachelor in beautiful Monument, Colorado, had exactly that same experience. "Almost immediately I lost the bloat," he says. And Bob McMicken, 51, from Lancaster, California, reported looking and feeling flatter "within days."

WEEK 2

SUDDEN, EFFORTLESS WEIGHT LOSS

When June Caron got on the scale at the beginning of week two, she was stunned: 6 pounds gone in the first seven days. "And the weight just keeps coming off," she says. The 55-year-old work control specialist from North Oxford,

Massachusetts, had begun to gain weight in her belly—the very thing that puts postmenopausal women at the same elevated risk for heart disease as men. It was a health crisis that needed attacking, but June had seen a lot of other weight-loss strategies fail—Weight Watchers, workout DVDs, you name it. "I've joined gyms but rarely stuck with them," she confesses. Now she finally had a plan that would help her manage not only her weight but also her health. Matt Brunner, a 43-year-old professor in Glenside, Pennsylvania, who had seen only mediocre results from past weight-loss plans, experienced the same thing: 7 pounds gone in just a week.

At the same time, back in Ohio, Martha Chesler was down 10 pounds within the first 10 days and starting to notice something else as well—her own health was improving measurably. At a checkup with her chiropractor, she discovered her heart was suddenly functioning much more efficiently. During a fitness test using a stationary cycle, when her heart rate would normally climb to 112 beats per minute within minutes of starting on the bike, she found an enormous change: "During the workout I could not raise my heart rate over 96 BPM! It was great to know good things were happening that I couldn't even see."

WEEK 3

OLD CLOTHES BECOME NEW AGAIN

Krista Kirk, 33, was always self-conscious about her belly, and when people started asking her if she was pregnant (she wasn't), she knew something had to change. Atkins, Nutrisystem—you name the plan, Krista can give the review: boring and ineffective. But after two weeks on the program, Krista discovered that her pants began to feel looser, her hips slimmed down—and she was finally able to dress in a way that reflected her true sense of style: "I'd avoided wearing high heels because the extra weight made my knees hurt so bad. I can actually wear my heels with confidence and without pain!"

In Pennsylvania, Matt Brunner was having the same experience. "My clothes got too big. My 'skinny' clothes all looked good again." And firefighter Morgan Minor was starting to see something she hadn't seen in years: her abs. "I had plateaued at 160 for over a month, and Zero Belly helped me lose more than 10 pounds in three weeks!"

WEEK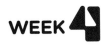

SCULPT YOUR NEW BODY

After a high-risk pregnancy during which she was unable to do more than walk, 38-year-old Jennie Joshi had been working hard to lose her baby weight. But the corporate sales trainer and mother of two simply couldn't get rid of her "pregnancy pooch." Low-carb, high-protein—you name the diet, Jennie had tried it. But the belly-specific, targeted approach of Zero Belly was different. She dropped 11 pounds in just about four weeks, but more important, she lost them where she wanted to lose them: "The pregnancy pooch is leaving!" she says. "I feel like the old pre-baby Jennie is back!"

Sticking to a weight-loss plan isn't easy for a working mom with two small children, and that's what impressed her about my program the most: The healthy recipes gave Jennie plenty of family-friendly options that even her foodie husband enjoyed. "Zero Belly is easy to follow regardless of life's demands. It's not a cleanse or a fad diet, it's a lifestyle."

And the fast results help keep you motivated. "I met a group of coworkers who hadn't seen me in a month, and they were all astonished at the differences they could see in me," says Fred Sparks, of Katy, Texas. "They wanted to know what I was doing."

It's at week four that the body-sculpting aspects of the protocol really begin to take effect. Beyond the flatter belly, most subjects also reported a leaner overall look. "My arms lost some of their flab, and my shoulders, biceps, and triceps tightened up," says Bryan. And the other side effects of the plan aren't bad, either. "My energy is at a very high level, whereas before Zero Belly I was feeling tired all the time," says June. "My skin and nails look better. I'm sleeping better. Everyone says I look much younger!"

WEEK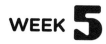

SAVE YOUR OWN LIFE

Katrina Bridges, of Bethalto, Illinois, wanted to lose weight and shrink her belly. But what she didn't know when she started Zero Belly was that she entered the test panel with a dramatically elevated risk of heart disease and diabetes.

In five weeks, that all changed. Katrina stripped off 12 pounds quickly, but more important, she shed 5 inches off her waistline, reducing her elevated risk of these diseases by a whopping 80 percent. And, she says, "I just felt like I had more overall strength throughout my body." The secret: Zero Belly drinks. "I loved the drinks," Katrina says. "They were all pretty easy, and I am sold on protein shakes."

Meanwhile, Martha Chesler was not only experiencing a healthier heart but something else: an end to her heartburn. "My acid reflux is under control, with minimum medication," she reports. And studies show heartburn isn't just an annoyance; like elevated belly fat, heartburn is a risk factor for certain types of cancer.

WEEK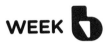

DRAMATIC CHANGES THAT LAST

I don't like to think of Zero Belly as a "weight loss" plan, although you'll lose a lot of weight. I like to think of it as a plan to shrink your waist and improve your life. So I get excited by stories like that of Kyle Cambridge of Peace River, Alberta, Canada, who lost 4 inches off his waist—and 25 pounds of fat—in just six weeks. "I even had to buy a new belt!" he says. "But the best was when Stacie [my wife] came up to me in the kitchen and gave me a hug. She laughed and smiled and said, 'I can wrap my hands around you again.'"

June Caron lost 4 inches off her waist in just six weeks. Fred Sparks stripped off 5 inches and 21 pounds of fat. Bob McMicken (down 24 pounds) and Bryan Wilson (19 pounds gone) both shed 6 inches. And Martha Chesler lost 21 pounds and 7 inches off her waist in less than 40 days. And they all remarked on how easy and effective the program was. "I love the Zero Belly drinks," says Bob. And June says, "It has been beyond comparison to any other diet or exercise program I have ever tried. I am never, ever hungry." These people discovered the amazing benefits of Zero Belly, and they did it without feeling hungry, tired, or overwhelmed.

I can't wait for you to join them!

WEIGHT-LOSS HACKS FROM THE ZERO BELLY TEST PANEL

A really great weight-loss plan is like a really great sport or game: It's got a set of rules that all players abide by—but that doesn't mean those rules can't be bent a little.

Like a poker player using her superior bluffing skills or a baseball pitcher rubbing a little dirt onto a shiny new ball, you can bring ideas into play that aren't in the rule book, per se—but can help you come out on top.

That's what many of the more than 500 folks who signed up for the original Zero Belly Test Panel did, and it helped some lose as much as 16 pounds in 14 days. By bending some of the traditional "diet rules," adapting the Zero Belly plan and the Zero Belly Smoothie recipes to their own needs and lifestyles, and playing some healthy mind games to make success their own, they lost the weight—and kept it off. Here are some of their weight-loss secrets.

WEIGHT-LOSS HACK #1

>Stop Using That Four-Letter Word

Diet, that is. When a fan site for the Zero Belly Diet sprang up on Facebook, I was more than gratified to discover that the fans themselves had decided to drop the word diet altogether and instead call their site "Zero Belly Way of Life."

When you "go on a diet," you're making the conscious decision that this is a temporary plan. But if you adopt a new way of living, it's yours forever. Breann Neal, 45, found that Zero Belly was the first plan that has helped her successfully deal with thyroid issues, and she lost 7 pounds and 3 inches off her waist in just two months. Even more dramatically, she says, "my husband has lost 20 pounds and is fitting into jeans that haven't fit him in three years.

"It's become a lifestyle for us," Breann explains. "We both feel so much healthier and have so much energy. My husband says this is the first diet he's ever been on that didn't feel like a diet."

Tell friends and family that you're "on a diet," and you'll have them focused on—and judging you by—your weight. But tell them you're making some lifestyle changes, and they'll start noticing other things, too. "I recently visited with a group of industry peers that I haven't seen for a year, and several of them commented that I looked younger than the last time they saw me," Breann says.

WEIGHT-LOSS HACK #2

>Use Your Family for Motivation

The allure of a flat belly, a leaner waist, maybe some new clothes—it's easy to get excited about a new weight-loss plan. But starting a diet or fitness program is easy. Sticking to it is a different issue.

And one of the reasons it can be hard to stay focused is that we tend to start programs for all the wrong reasons. A 2014 study in the journal *Body Image* looked at 321 college-age women and found that, long term, those who exercised primarily for appearance-based reasons had a harder time sticking to their fitness plans than those who worked out to maintain their health. Instead of motivating yourself with dreams of rippled abs, try posting photos of the people who love and depend on you by your fridge or computer—and remember, they're the ones who really benefit when you lose weight.

WEIGHT-LOSS HACK #3

>Stop Being Hungry!

One of the hardest concepts for some folks to get their heads around is the idea of losing weight without having to feel hungry all the time.

"Before Zero Belly I thought I was doing well by skipping meals, eating a salad for lunch every now and then, and walking long distances to try to control my weight," says Isabel Fiolek, age 56. "It wasn't working; I was slowly gaining weight and adding inches. Zero Belly taught me to eat smaller meals throughout the day and to eat much healthier food. I was on Zero Belly for six weeks and lost 13 pounds—and I've kept it off for a year."

And Jason Johnson, age 40, found that denying himself food did nothing more than deny him success. "I always felt that in order to eat healthy, it meant I had to be used to being hungry all the time. But by focusing on the foods outlined by Zero Belly, I have discovered that I can eat great-tasting food, not feel hungry, and lose weight."

What worked for our test panel was making sure the participants always had a Zero Belly snack in hand, just in case. Craving food and not knowing what to eat is like finding yourself in a minefield without a map. In fact, Dutch researchers posed a group of test subjects a series of questions like, "If you're hungry at 4 p.m., then...what?" Those who had an answer ("I'll snack on some almonds") were more successful at losing weight than those who didn't.

WEIGHT-LOSS HACK #4

>Follow Your Moods

Part of the virtue of Zero Belly Smoothies is that they fill you with foods that promote a healthy gut biome. Researchers in Ireland found that mice treated with gut-healthy probiotics suffered less stress, anxiety, and depression-related behavior—which makes sense, since 90 percent of our stores of the feel-good hormone serotonin are actually located not in the brain but in the belly. And Zero Belly Smoothie nutrients like piperine (from fresh black pepper), omega-3 fatty acids (from chia and flax), and folate (from leafy greens and peanuts) have been linked directly to a reduced risk of depression. If you're blue, it may be a signal that the nutrients in your diet are out of balance.

"I've noticed that after I eat food that is not as healthy for me, I tend to not feel as well as I do when I'm eating nutrient-dense foods," says Jason. "It's an eye-opener to how rundown I was feeling every day of my life, now that I'm one of those (probably) annoying good-mood people.

"I have been doing Zero Belly for five weeks, and I've lost 18 pounds and 3 inches off my waist," Jason continues. "But the biggest change is this energy and mood shift," which he says happened on day three of the plan. "I suddenly felt happy, almost euphoric, and my body told me I should just get up and start walking. I know it sounds corny, but it's true."

WEIGHT-LOSS HACK #5
>Freeze Up Your Time

Simple, immediate, and stress-free. That's what I want Zero Belly to be: a plan that pays off for you quickly, without a lot of hassle and effort. And a key part of that plan is the simple, immediate, and stress-free recipes for Zero Belly Smoothies—plant-based concoctions that are high in the three essential macronutrients of the plan: protein, fiber, and healthy fats.

But whipping up a smoothie isn't always convenient, especially if your mornings are hectic and your office doesn't have a blender-friendly kitchen. That's why I loved this hack from Facebook fan Theresa Nihan Case, who has a simple solution: "I make my shakes the night before and freeze them in mason jars. Then pack them in a cooler bag with an ice pack. Just take them out a few hours before you want to drink." An added benefit, according to Theresa: "Frozen, you drink it way slower, keeping you full longer." To make blending easier, always add your liquids first, then the protein and fruit; experiment with how much liquid you need to find the perfect consistency for you.

5-MINUTE FLAT-BELLY TIP:

CALL MERLOT THE MAGICIAN

Have a glass of red wine or two a week. It could help you burn fat better, according to a 2015 study in *Nutritional Biochemistry*. Over a 10-week trial, mice that got the human equivalent of about 1½ cups of red grapes a day accumulated less abdominal fat and had lower blood sugar than those that didn't—even though both sets of furry subjects were being fed high-fat diets. In fact, the ellagic acid in the grapes lowered the fat mice's blood sugar to nearly the same levels as those of lean, normally fed mice.

Red wine is the best possible source of a micronutrient called resveratrol, which works on the genes responsible for obesity and liver steatosis—essentially, belly fat that forms around your liver. That's because resveratrol is found primarily in the skin of grapes, and the alcohol in wine draws the resveratrol out of the skins, creating a concentrated dose that's greater than what's found in just grape juice. (You know how, if you leave a splash of wine sitting in a glass overnight, you get a flaky burgundy deposit at the bottom? That's resveratrol.)

5 BEST VEGETABLES FOR MUSCLES AND STRENGTH

When it comes to building lean, belly-fat-burning muscle, getting enough protein is as fundamental as advertised. But if you're chronically bypassing the produce aisle for the meat case in your quest for progress, you're selling yourself short. Certain vegetables are packed with nutrients that have demonstrated muscle- and strength-boosting properties. They deserve a place on your plate, pronto.

BEETS

The mild-mannered root vegetable is nature's steroid. A number of studies have shown that consuming the carpet-staining vegetable can improve your athletic performance. Athletes who drank beet juice experienced a 38 percent increase in blood flow to muscles, particularly "fast twitch" muscles that affect bursts of speed and strength, according to a study conducted at Kansas State University. Another study published in the *Journal of the Academy of Nutrition and Dietetics* found that runners who ate baked beets before a 5K race ran 5 percent faster. The secret weapon: nitrates, a natural chemical that increases endurance and lowers blood pressure.

SPINACH

Downing iron is as important as lifting it—the mineral is crucial to building muscle and strength, and spinach is the dietary MVP. According to the United States Department of Agriculture, a 180-gram serving of boiled spinach has 6.43 milligrams of iron—more than a 6-ounce piece of hamburger. The leafy green is also an excellent source of magnesium, a mineral that's essential to muscle development, energy production, and carb metabolism. Two studies have found that levels of testosterone (and muscle strength) are directly correlated to the levels of magnesium in the body. Other good veggie sources of magnesium: radishes, soybeans, and chard.

SWEET POTATOES

There's a reason bodybuilders scarf these with their chicken breasts: They're one of the cleanest sources of fuel available. High in fiber and carbs (4 grams and 27 grams per serving, respectively), the vibrant tubers have a low glycemic index, meaning they burn slowly, providing a long-term source of energy that helps you power up after a workout and recover your stores of muscle glycogen afterward. The fiber keeps you fuller longer, helping prevent the overeating that'll shatter your dreams of shredded abs. Bonus: One cup of sweet potato cubes has four times your RDA of vitamin A, which helps your body synthesize protein.

MUSHROOMS

One variety of this veggie is the No. 1 vegetable source of vitamin D, which researchers have begun to find may play a role in muscle building. In a recent study published in the journal *Medicine & Science in Sports & Exercise*, researchers measured the leg and arm strength of 419 men and women and tested their vitamin D levels; they found that participants with higher levels of D were stronger. A separate analysis of 30 studies involving 5,615 people found that D supplementation was positively associated with muscle strength. The best mushroom to buy is maitake, aka "hen of the woods." One cup provides three times your daily allowance of D! Other varieties that are D-rich: chanterelle, morel, and shiitake.

PEPPERS

Green, red, or yellow all mean go—peppers are the vegetable with the highest amount of vitamin C, which helps burn fat and turn carbs into fuel. In a study published in *The American Journal of Clinical Nutrition*, researchers found that muscle tissue drinks up vitamin C, helping it process carnitine, a fatty acid that's essential to muscle growth and recovery. Just half a cup of peppers provides 300 percent of your recommended daily intake of C.

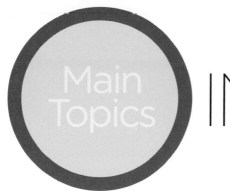

Main Topics

INDEX

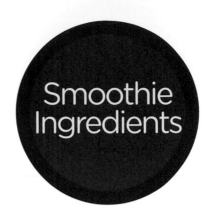

Smoothie Ingredients

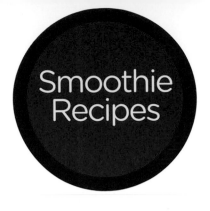

Smoothie Recipes

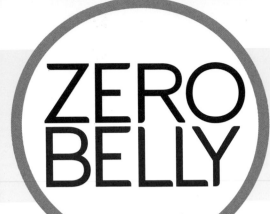

ZERO BELLY

The Revolutionary Plan to Turn Off Your Fat Genes and Lose Up to 16 Pounds in 14 Days!

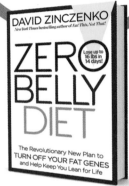

THE *NEW YORK TIMES* BESTSELLER!

Turn off your fat genes, strip away belly fat and finally attain the lean, strong, healthy body you've always wanted.

Get daily updates on weight-loss tricks, belly fat news and amazing recipes.

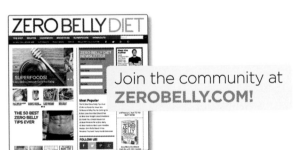

Join the community at **ZEROBELLY.COM!**

Metabolism-boosting breakfasts. Flat-belly lunches. Fat-melting dinners. To shed belly flab— while eating the foods you love— turn to the 150+ recipes in **THE ZERO BELLY COOKBOOK!**

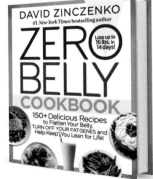